Sexuality
and Serious Mental Illness

Chronic Mental Illness

Sexuality
and Serious Mental Illness

Edited by

Peter F. Buckley, MD
Case Western Reserve University
Cleveland, Ohio, USA

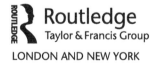

Routledge
Taylor & Francis Group

LONDON AND NEW YORK

First published 1999 by Harwood Academic Publishers

Published 2021 by Routledge
2 Park Square, Milton Park, Abingdon, Oxon OX14 4RN
605 Third Avenue, New York, NY 10017

Routledge is an imprint of the Taylor & Francis Group, an informa business

British Library Cataloguing in Publication Data

Sexuality and serious mental illness. – (Chronic mental
   illness ; v. 7 – ISSN 1066-7407)
   1. Mentally ill – Sexual behavior
   I. Buckley, Peter F.
   362.2

ISBN 13: 978-90-5702-598-3 (hbk)
ISBN 13: 978-11-3801-003-1 (pbk)

CONTENTS

INTRODUCTION TO THE SERIES

This series on chronic mental illness is a result of both the success and failure of our efforts over the past thirty years to provide better treatment, rehabilitation and care for persons suffering from severe and persistent mental illnesses. The failure is obvious to all who walk our cities' streets, use our libraries or pass through our transportation terminals. The success is found in the enormous boost of interest in service to, research on and teaching about treatment, rehabilitation and care of those persons who, in Leona Bachrach's definition, "are, have been, or might have been, but for the deinstitutionalization movement, on the rolls of long-term mental institutions, especially state hospitals."

The first book in our modern era devoted to the subject was that by Richard Lamb in 1976, *Community Survival for Long-Term Patients.* Shortly thereafter, Leona Bachrach's unique study "Deinstitutionalization: An Analytical Review and Sociological Perspective" was published. In 1978, the American Psychiatric Association hosted a meeting on the problem that resulted in the publication *The Chronic Mental Patient.* This effort in turn spawned several texts dealing with increasingly specialized areas: *The Chronic Mentally Ill: Treatment, Programs, Systems* and *Chronic Mental Illness in Children and Adolescents,* both by John Looney; and *The Chronic Mental Patient/II* by Walter Menninger and Gerald Hannah.

Now, however, there are a host of publications devoted to various portions of the problem, e.g., the homeless mentally ill, rehabilitation of the mentally ill, families of the mentally ill and so on. The amount of research and experience now that can be conveyed to a wide population of caregivers is exponentially greater than it was in 1955, the year that deinstitutionalization began.

This series will cover:

— types of intervention, e.g., psychopharmacology, psychotherapy, case management, social and vocational rehabilitation and mobile and home treatment;
— settings, e.g., hospitals, ambulatory settings, nursing homes, correctional facilities and shelters;
— specific populations, e.g., alcohol and drug abusers, the homeless and those dually diagnosed;

— special issues, e.g., family intervention, psychoeducation, policy/ financing, non-compliance, forensic, cross-cultural and systems issues.

I am indebted to our hard-working editorial board as well as to our editors and authors, many of whom are involved in both activities.

This latest volume deals with a subject that no one has tackled to date and that provokes much concern: sexuality in the seriously mentally ill. It is comprehensive and practical, helpful yet academically rigorous, and useful to so many of us in the field who have struggled with these issues. Its editor and authors are able to communicate the many complex facets of this problem engagingly.

Future books in the series will deal with legal issues, housing and residential care, the chronicity of substance abuse, inpatient care, ethics and psychopharmacology — all as related to the treatment, care and rehabilitation of the chronic mentally ill. I hope you'll look forward to them as much as I do.

John A. Talbott, MD

PREFACE

Sexual activity among persons with serious mental illness is an issue of clinical, social and legal concern. Accurate delineation of the prevalence of sexual activity in this population is obfuscated by misconceptions and by the intensely personal nature of this behavior. Moreover, sexuality in persons with serious mental illness has traditionally been considered an uncommon occurrence because of anhedonia, psychosocial impairment and medication-induced sexual dysfunction. Recent research challenges these assumptions and suggests that as many as 50% of those with serious mental illness will engage in sexual activity. Individuals may become sexually active as an expression of normal sexuality, or as a consequence of psychotic symptoms. Additionally, the institutional subculture may foster such behavior. This volume provides a timely and authoritative overview of critical aspects of this important topic.

The book is timely because of several developments in mental health. First, the current culture of psychiatric consumerism promotes personal autonomy and the expression of fundamental human rights, including individual choice among persons with mental illness. Second, the allied movement of advocacy places emphasis on patient involvement in their care and on the importance of respect and human dignity. Third, the recovery model stresses the personal experiences of patients with mental illness, including the capacity for personal fulfillment and sexuality. This model holds primacy in current perspectives on rehabilitation for persons with mental illness. Fundamentally, the recovery model views normalization as the key approach for success. Fourth, the array of new and more efficacious treatments are resulting in improved outcomes and a greater likelihood that patients will achieve satisfying life experiences, one of which is intimacy. At the same time, we have become increasingly preoccupied with the issues of competency, informed consent and the legal obligations of the mental health system to protect vulnerable individuals and the community at large.

In the opening chapter, Dr. Buckley and colleagues review the epidemiology, patterns and clinical characteristics of sexual activity among persons with severe mental illness, with respect to both hospital and community settings. In the second chapter, Dr. Deegan, a psychiatric consumer and nationally known advocate, discusses these complex issues from the patient's perspective. She describes human sexuality as a component of the recovery process for persons with mental illness. In considering sexuality as a human right, Dr. Noffsinger (chapter 3) details the legal literature, including available information on litigation. He discusses how this right is further upheld under the Americans with Disabilities Act of 1990 and explores the forensic aspects of sexuality among patients with mental illness, including competency assessments.

In tandem with respect for patient rights and privacy, hospital administrators must protect vulnerable individuals under their care and must also uphold official and social policies. In chapter 4 Dr. Buckley et al. describe these dilemmas and provide information on the management of sexual incidents and on the content of sexual policies in state facilities. The following chapter by Dr. Welch and colleagues provides a detailed account of an innovative approach to developing and implementing a policy for consensual sex among inpatients. They describe their experiences with this policy, its strengths and weaknesses that became evident upon implementation, and they offer practical suggestions for developing a successful policy.

Despite the importance of this topic, relatively little attention has been given to developing psychosexual education programs. In their chapter (chapter 6), Dr. Kopelowicz and colleagues review the literature and describe the components of a new psychosexual module they have recently developed. Their training module focuses on intimacy and sexual relationships. This chapter describes in detail how this module can be used to inform and modify sexual attitudes and practices in this patient group.

Much of the current interest in sexuality and mental illness stems from recent research on HIV risk among persons with serious mental illness. Drs. McKinnon and Cournos, leading contributors to this literature, provide a detailed account in chapter 7 of the epidemiology of HIV in persons with mental illness, its attendant risk factors and its impact upon psychiatric illness.

Dr. Rosenberg et al. (chapter 8) then address a largely under-appreciated and under-researched aspect of pre-morbid development in individuals with serious mental illness. Their chapter examines the extent and implications for management of sexual trauma and re-victimization in persons with serious mental illness.

In chapter 9, Dr. Milner and colleagues highlight the impact of various classes of psychotropic medications upon sexual functioning among individuals with serious mental illness. The different mechanisms that contribute to sexual dysfunction are described, with some emphasis on the pattern of dysfunction now observed with the use of novel anti-psychotic medications. Practical advice is given on interventions to ameliorate such dysfunction. From a different but complementary vantage point, Dr. McElroy et al. (chapter 10) describe contemporary pharmacological approaches to the management of sexual deviancy and related behaviors. They apply this to current findings on the neurobiology of impulse control and sexual arousal.

The concluding chapter by Drs. Buckley and Gutheil proposes that sexuality and mental illness be conceptualized as one component of the larger topic of stigmatization of the mentally ill. They point out that, while hospital administrators struggle with upholding conflicting responsibilities in this realm, the law itself is internally consistent with respect to freedom and autonomy.

Because of its topic and diversity of chapters, it is hoped that this book will be useful to a broad audience. Clinicians of all disciplines (nursing, psychology, psychiatry, rehabilitation, social work) should find it a source of practical information and guidance in addressing this topic in everyday practice. Administrators and clinicians are provided with a full discourse on the ethical and practical complexities of developing policies sensitive to this issue. Moreover, its broader legal and social contexts are emphasized. Social scientists and interested attorneys may appreciate the breadth of review within these pages. It should also be evident that this book comes to the shelves at a time in service delivery when the rights and interests of persons with mental illness and their relatives are at a premium. It is hoped that the information contained here will be helpful to individuals and their relatives who wish to promote greater discussion of these issues.

This volume, which brings together the collective knowledge and experience of experts, reflects the current level of understanding of the complexities of sexual activity among persons with serious mental illness. The contributors are to be sincerely thanked for their insights and guidance.

CONTRIBUTORS

Peter F. Buckley, MD, Medical Director, Northcoast Behavioral Healthcare System, Northfield, Ohio; Associate Professor of Psychiatry, Case Western Reserve University, Cleveland, Ohio.

Mitch Caine, PhD, Clinical Psychologist, Los Angeles County Department of Mental Health, Los Angeles, California.

Gerrit W. Clements, BA, LLB, Special Health Consultant, Ministry of Health and Ministry Responsible for Seniors; Adjunct Professor, School of Health Information Science, Faculty of Human and Social Development, University of Victoria, British Columbia.

Francine Cournos, MD, Director, Washington Heights Community Service, New York State Psychiatric Institute, New York, New York.

Patricia E. Deegan, PhD, Director of Training and Education, National Empowerment Center, Lawrence, Massachusetts.

Timothy Florence, MD, Clinical Instructor, University of Michigan Hospital, Ann Arbor, Michigan.

Lee Friedman, PhD, Assistant Professor of Psychiatry, Case Western Reserve University, Cleveland, Ohio.

George Gintoli, MS, Chief Executive Officer, Northcoast Behavioral Healthcare System, Northfield, Ohio.

Lisa A. Goodman, PhD, Assistant Professor, Department of Psychology, University of Maryland, College Park.

Thomas G. Gutheil, MD, Professor of Psychiatry, Harvard Medical School, Boston, Massachusetts.

Michael Hogan, PhD, Director, Ohio Department of Mental Health, Columbus, Ohio.

Jodi Hyde, BA, Research Assistant, Case Western Reserve University, Cleveland, Ohio.

Paul E. Keck, Jr., MD, Professor of Psychiatry and Vice Chairman for Research, Department of Psychiatry, University of Cincinnati College of Medicine, Cincinnati, Ohio.

Alex Kopelowicz, MD, Assistant Professor of Psychiatry, School of Medicine, University of California, Los Angeles, California; Medical Director, San Fernando Mental Health Center, Mission Hills, California.

Robert G. Mangano, BS, Research Associate, Department of Psychiatry and Biobehavioral Sciences, University of California, Los Angeles, California.

Susan L. McElroy, MD, Professor of Psychiatry, University of Cincinnati, Cincinnati, Ohio.

Karen McKinnon, MA, Project Director, Columbia University HIV Mental Health Training Project, College of Physicians and Surgeons, Department of Psychiatry, Columbia University, New York, New York.

Karen Milner, MD, Clinical Assistant Professor, Director of Psychiatric Emergency Room, University of Michigan Hospital, Ann Arbor, Michigan.

Margaret E. Moreau, PhD, Senior Psychologist, Program Evaluation Services, Riverview Hospital, Port Coquitlan, British Columbia.

Kim T. Mueser, PhD, Professor, Department of Psychiatry and Community & Family Medicine, Dartmouth Medical School, Hanover, New Hampshire; Senior Research Professor, New Hampshire-Dartmouth Psychiatric Research Center, Concord and Lebanon, New Hampshire.

Stephen G. Noffsinger, MD, Director of Forensic Psychiatry, Northcoast Behavioral Healthcare System, Northfield, Ohio; Assistant Professor of Psychiatry, Case Western Reserve University, Cleveland, Ohio.

Tricia Robben, BA, Research Assistant, Case Western Reserve University, Cleveland, Ohio.

Stanley D. Rosenberg, PhD, Professor of Psychiatry, Dartmouth Medical School, Lebanon, New Hampshire.

Cesar A. Soutullo, MD, Child and Adolescent Psychiatry Fellow, Division of Child and Adolescent Psychiatry and Biological Psychiatry Program, Department of Psychiatry, University of Cincinnati College of Medicine, Cincinnati, Ohio.

Dale P. Svendsen, MD, Medical Director, Ohio Department of Mental Health, Columbus, Ohio.

Rajiv Tandon, MD, Associate Professor of Psychiatry, University of Michigan, Ann Arbor, Michigan.

Kim M. Thompson, MA, Graduate Assistant II, Department of Psychology, University of Maryland, College Park.

Oladapo Tomori, MD, Clinical Instructor, University of Michigan, Ann Arbor, Michigan.

Steven J. Welch, PhD, Chairperson of the Taskforce on Patient Sexuality, Department of Psychology, Riverview Hospital, Port Coquitlan, British Columbia.

1

Sexual Behavior in Persons with Serious Mental Illness: Patterns and Clinical Correlates

PETER F. BUCKLEY, TRICIA ROBBEN, LEE FRIEDMAN and JODI HYDE

The sexual practices of persons with serious mental illness raise important clinical, social and legal concerns. Yet, in spite of the seriousness of this topic, there is relatively little systematic information on the extent and pattern of sexual activity in this population. This chapter provides an account of the current knowledge of this issue viewed in the context of normative sexual practices in the population at large and sexual activity among patients with other psychiatric disorders.

Normative Sexual Practices

Few aspects of human activity evoke the interest of the media and popular press as much as sexuality. We are bombarded with television and magazine reports of sexual interests, preferences, and lifestyles in the 1990s. However, surprisingly, and in contrast to this voluminous lay literature, epidemiological research on the normative expression of sexuality is relatively scant. Such information is important and is required to inform and guide public health policy regarding HIV infection and other sexually transmitted diseases. Epidemiological information on sexuality in the general population is also of direct importance to psychiatry as it provides the backdrop to evaluating sexual impulsivity, sexual deviancy, sexual dysfunction and sexuality in clinical practice.

Several, well-conducted epidemiological surveys have recently addressed this issue. In a British random-sample survey of 18,876 males and females (age range 16–59) that was conducted during 1990–1991 (Johnson *et al.*, 1992), it was observed that 8.2% of males and 4.8% of females reported having 2 or more heterosexual partners in the previous year. Sexual activity was increased among those who were unmarried, of higher social class, and who had first intercourse before age 16. While just over 60% of males reported any lifetime homosexual experience, 3.6% of males had a current homosexual partner. Results from a French study broadly endorsed these findings and emphasized that only 59% of males had used condoms in the last year (ACSF, 1992). The median age at first intercourse was 17 years for men and 18 years for women. Lifetime rates of homosexual intercourse were recorded at 4.1% for males and 2.6% for females, although the majority (approximately 80%) of these people had bisexual experiences. Seidman and Reider (1994) conducted a comprehensive review of epidemiological data on human sexuality collected from several American public health surveys. Their findings are summarized in Table 1.1. In brief, they highlighted that the overwhelming majority of adolescents are sexually active by age 19. Adolescents experience multiple, serial sexual relationships. Young adults show a similar pattern, while older adults tend towards monogamy and a declining frequency of sexual activity. Although estimates vary, some 3% of males are exclusively homosexual and a similar percentage have bisexual practices (Seidman and Reider, 1994).

Assessment of Sexual Behavior

As stated above, sexual preferences and practices are highly personal and emotive issues. There is no simple or best manner to assess sexual practices among persons with mental illness. Approaches to assessing sexual behavior vary widely, both in their sensitivity and degree of intrusion upon patient privacy (see Table 1.2). Approaches used in studies of sexual behavior among persons with serious mental illness are highlighted in Tables 1.3 and 1.4.

Sexual attitudes may be explored by way of self-report questionnaires. These have the advantage of being minimally intrusive and, accordingly, may encourage candid disclosure of personal information. However, these questionnaires are difficult to construct and require the use of language that is clear and neutral. Also, they must avoid being either too technical (vivid descriptions may be offensive) or overly-vernacular. Also, information derived from a self-report questionnaire may be unreliable and is open to all the vicissitudes of survey research (Johnson *et al.*, 1992); this is compounded by the

Table 1.1. Representative Data on Sexual Activity Among American Men and Women.[1, 2, 3]

	% Sexually Active	2 or More Partners	Frequency of Intercourse
Aged 15-19			
Females	66% - 75%	46%	39.5% females, 53.5% males
Males	79% - 86%	40.5%	had sex during the preceding 3 months
Aged 19-24			
Females	81%	31%	35% females, 28% males had
Males	84%	56%	intercourse more than 10 times a month
Aged 25+			
Females	- - -	66%	58% females, 43% males had
Males	91%	80%	intercourse more than once a week

[1]Data derived from several epidemiological studies – see Seidman and Reider (1994).
[2]Sexual activity refers to heterosexual intercourse.
[3]1-6% males engaged in homosexual activity; data for females was not given.

possible influences of psychiatric symptoms and cognitive impairment. Review of clinical records is perhaps the least intrusive approach but this is of most dubious value since clinicians rarely document (at all) the sexual experiences of inpatients. Inquiring staff directly about their observations of the sexual behavior of patients is an approach best used as a collateral rather than primary source of information. It is difficult to obtain detailed information from staff and they may be genuinely unaware of the patient's lifestyle in the community. Moreover, the information is likely to be influenced by that individual's sexual attitudes. On the other hand, collateral history from staff can be of great assistance in instances of alleged sexual assault between inpatients or when a psychotic patient with sexual preoccupations makes an erroneous allegation of sexual misconduct by staff on the unit.

Clinical assessment of patients requires attention to their sexual history. However, this aspect of the psychiatric evaluation is underemphasized and clinicians frequently obtain (at best) only superficial and cursory information. This point is well emphasized in other chapters in this book. More recent studies of high-risk sexual behavior among persons with serious mental illness (see Tables 1.3

Table 1.2. Approaches to the Assessment for Sexual Behavior Among Mentally Ill Patients.

Method	Strengths	Weaknesses
Self-report	protects privacy; may allow for individual comments; brief	reliability unknown without collateral; patient may be confused and misinterpret information
Medical chart review	not intrusive, combines patient report and (multiple) staff observations	sexual histories often incomplete; staff rarely document sexual behavior
Staff observation/ questionnaire	direct observation; not intrusive to patient	staff perceptions may be inaccurate; personal mores may bias data
Patient interview	source information; may access sensitive issues	patient may not disclose personal information; clinicians may be unskilled in questioning sexual matters
Structure patient interview/ questionnaire	more detailed information scale may have established reliability	may be too detailed to administer; time consuming
Patient physical examination	objective; of medicolegal importance	intrusive; rarely appropriate; information obtained may not be specific
Laboratory testing – semen testing – STD testing – HIV testing	objective; useful in prevention of spread/minimizing risk to population	intrusive; major ethical considerations

Table 1.3. Representative Studies of Sexual Activity in Patients with Schizophrenia.

	Assessment Method	Period of Observation	Patient/ Control Sample	Site	Sexually Active	Sexual Relations Comments
Akhtar (77)	SI	two years	34	inpatient	3.1%	94% of encounters were heterosexual
Modestin (81)	observation	one year	16	inpatient	1.5%	100% heterosexual of sexual activity
Lyketsos (83)	PQ	inpatient	113/106	inpatient	N.S.	87% males, 42% females had sexual dysfunction associated with psychotropic meds
Friedman (84)	SQ, SSPI	life time	20/15	community	N.S.	60% female patients (13.4% controls) never experienced orgasm
Rozensky (84)	PQ	life time	61	community	80%	18.5 mean age at first intercourse; 16% homosexual
Raboch (86)	SPI	six years	20/101	community	N.S.	slower sexual development among female patients (versus controls)
Baker (91)	SPI	one year	23	community	78%	57% of adolescent females reported high-risk sexual behaviors
Kelly (92)	PQ	one year	60	community	62%	42% males, 19% females had multiple partners/infrequent condom use
Volvaka (92)	PQ	one year	476	community	N.S.	14.4% high-risk patients HIV positive
Cournos (93)	SPI	six months	95	community	57.8%	9.8% patients use condoms; 18.5% patients had homosexual experiences
Diclemente (93)	SPI	15 months	76/802	community	53%	mean age of first intercourse = 11.4 years; 20% had homosexual experience
Cournos (94)	SPI	six months	95	community	44%	22% had some (lifetime) homosexual experience

Buckley *et al.*

Table 1.3. (Continued)

	Assessment Method	Period of Observation	Patient/ Control Sample	Site	Sexually Active	Sexual Relations Comments
Kalichman (94)	SPI	one year	95	community	54%	18% received drugs/money for sex; 27% had multiple partners
McDermott (94)	PQ, SPI	six months	61/32	community	N.S.	22% had homosexual experience; psychiatric patients frequency of intercourse for a month is similar (9.5 times versus 9.8 control subjects)
Susser (95)	SSPI	two years	122	community	53%	86% heterosexuals; 30.7% homosexuals (includes bisexuals); half of sexually active men didn't use a condom with a non-monogamous partner
Chuang (96)	PQ	one year	151	community	51.7%	25% thought one unsafe sexual contact would not have them vulnerable to AIDS; 33% do not insist on condom use
Coverdale (97)	PQ	one year	66/66	community	55.4%	patients were more likely than controls to have coerced sex

PQ = patient questionnaire
SQ = staff questionnaire
SI = staff interview
SSPI = semi-structured interview
SPI = structured patient interview
N.S. = not specified

Table 1.4. Representative Studies that Detail the Pattern of Sexual Activity Among Patients with Serious Mental Illness.

	Sexually Active	Relationships Monog/Multiple	Sex in Exchange for Money/Goods	Use of Contraception	Alcohol/Drug Abuse	Treatment for STD's	Masturbation
Rozensky (84)	80%	N.S.	N.S.	23%	N.S.	N.S.	88%
Baker (91)	78%	N.S.	N.S.	17%	30%	17%	N.S.
Kelly (92)	62%	42%m 19%f	13% N.S.	15%	91%	33%	N.S.
Cournos (93)	57.8%	44.6%	N.S.	9.8%	N.S.	N.S.	N.S.
Diclemente (93)	53%	N.S.	15%	23%	9%	15%	N.S.
Cournos (94)	44%	62%	50%	9.8%	45%	N.S.	N.S.
Kalichman (94)	54%	27%	18%	24%	<50%	32%	N.S.
Susser (95)	53%	21%	25%	24%	65%	N.S.	N.S.
Chaung (96)	51.7%	17.4%	6.7%	N.S.	N.S.	5.4%	N.S.
Coverdale (87)	55.4%	36.4%	2.9%	N.S.	N.S.	18%	N.S.

N.S. = Not Specified

and 1.4) demonstrate that is possible through careful interviewing to elicit reliable information on sensitive, sexual details. Moreover, once questions are appropriately phrased, persons with mental illness do not mind (and in fact anticipate) being questioned about intimacy (Crawford and Shaw, 1998; also see Deegan, this volume). The quality of information is dependent upon the frankness of the patient, the context of the assessment, the quality of the therapeutic alliance, and the skill of the clinician. For research purposes, the use of structured interviews can help to provide more direct and exact information on sexual practices in a manner that is reproducible and quantifiable across different studies. Several useful scales have been published. Volavka and colleagues (1992) also reported good reliability for a 13-item screening questionnaire, the Risk Behavior Questionnaire. Burke and colleagues (1994) described a structured interview to evaluate sexual function in male patients with schizophrenia. Carmen and Brady (1990) have described a checklist for assessing sexual history and risk of HIV. Several other studies cited in Tables 1.3 and 1.4 used other questionnaires developed to assess patient sexuality (details on specific questions are not given but the primary authors indicate that the scale is available upon request).

Finally, physical examination and relevant testing may be appropriate and helpful in a minority of cases (e.g., when medicolegal concerns arise; [also see Noffsinger, this volume]). Examinations should be performed (after appropriate consent is obtained) by a physician other than the attending psychiatrist. HIV testing is another important component of the patient evaluation, although such testing is fraught with serious ethical considerations (Grassi, 1996).

Accurate detection of sexual behavior among patients may be enhanced by staff who are appropriately trained to assess and manage this issue. This is a generally neglected area for staff training. Staff are often bewildered when confronted with issues of patient sexuality (Mossman *et al.*, 1997). Staff may have inconsistent and ill-formed personal values regarding sexuality and they differ widely in their level of knowledge about human sexuality and its health consequences (Civic *et al.*, 1993). Staff require explicit information and training about aspects of sexuality and their implications for care of psychiatric patients. Staff need to learn how to take a detailed sexual history and elicit personal details in a non-threatening, open manner. Such training should occur early in the health professional's career since this will emphasize its importance and counter historical misconceptions. At present, medical students and residents are not taught a format for acquiring information on sexual activity.

Misconceptions Regarding Sex and Serious Mental Illness

The stereotypic impression is that persons with serious mental illness are either asexual or have bizarre sexual experiences. The former impression was supported by earlier studies showing a very low rate of sexual activity among patients. For example, Modestin found only 9 instances of sexual intercourse over a one year period by 16 of 1,060 patients (Modestin, 1981). Similarly, Akhtar and colleagues could only identify 34 of 1,120 inpatients who had been 'sexually explicit' (defined as intercourse, masturbation, or fondling) during a 2-year period (Akhtar *et al.*, 1977). Reports of sexuality among inpatients were uncommon and the prevailing attitude (even more than today) was to dismiss the issue and conclude that persons with serious mental illness were incapable of meaningful sexual relationships. At the same time, evidence of patient sexuality was viewed in psychodynamic terms: "the onset of schizophrenia often causes a release of sexual impulses, experienced initially as obsessional urges, preoccupations and vague bodily sensations. This upsurge often results in delusions, elaborate hallucinatory phenomena, and sexual acting out. The form such release takes varies with the individual's psychodynamic constellation, as well as the degree of regression" (Akhtar and Thompson, 1980). Sexual aberrancy was closely equated to mental disturbance: "self-induced genital injury and autocastration are almost pathognomonic of schizophrenia" (Akhtar and Thompson, 1980). Moreover, it was hypothesized that sexual excesses, masturbation and bizarre activities could induce psychosis (Nesteros *et al.*, 1981). In a survey of U.S. psychiatrists and patients (Pinderhughes *et al.*, 1972), 66% of psychiatrists considered sexual activity a contributory factor to psychosis. Thirty-three percent of psychiatrists and a similar number of patients believed that sexual activity was detrimental to recovery from mental illness. Nesteros and colleagues (1981) conducted an extensive literature search which revealed only four clinical studies published between 1966 and 1980. In their own study (Nesteros *et al.*, 1981), they reported that only eight percent of male patients were sexually active before the onset of their illness and only two percent in the year prior to the survey (compared with 58% of control subjects); heterosexual and autoerotic (masturbatory) activity predominated. Fourteen percent of patients reported that they had never engaged in any kind of sexual activity or ideation. Additionally, 22% of patients reported impotence, 19% had retarded ejaculation and 32% were unable to ejaculate.

The term "neglect and psychiatrization" was coined to describe the response of professionals to sexuality among persons with mental illness (Vandereycken, 1993). Psychiatrists infrequently inquire about sexual side-effects of medication in their patients, implying that this is an unimportant concern. Patients' sexual lives were considered disturbed and should be a treatable consequence of their mental disorder. Vandereycken argued that professional staff were confused by patient sexuality and that their medicalized stance thereby avoided confronting the issue. This point is further emphasized in the chapter by Dr. Deegan in this book.

More recent prevalence studies estimating sexual activity among persons with serious mental illness vary widely depending upon the method of assessment, the patient population (age, gender, ethnic and diagnostic composition) and the definition of sexual activity (see Tables 1.1–1.3); the latter may range from intimate personal contact to sexual intercourse. Such variability still impedes our understanding of the context of sexuality and mental illness.

Sexual Activity Among Outpatients

The spread of HIV infection in the 1980s and the specter of AIDS focused attention on the sexual activity of persons with serious mental illness, leading to a spate of studies examining high-risk sexual behavior (see Table 1.3 and 1.4). Findings from these studies are salutary and contrast starkly with historical perspectives of asexuality. These studies confirm that (in spite of the disabilities of the illness) rates of sexual activity of approximately 50% are observed among out patients with schizophrenia. The study by Cournos and colleagues (1994) is illustrative: using the Sexual Risk Behavior Assessment (SERBAS); McKinnon et al., 1993, they reported that 42 of 95 patients (44%) with a diagnosis of schizophrenia had been sexually active in the preceding 6 months; sexual activity primarily involved heterosexual intercourse. Sixty-two percent of sexually active persons had multiple partners and 12% had intercourse with a partner who was either HIV positive or had injected drugs. Other studies (Diclemente and Ponton, 1993; Kelly, 1992) confirm these observations. Diclemente and Ponton reported that 53% adolescents with psychiatric disorders (diagnoses were not specified) were sexually active in contrast with a rate of 29% among the control group of 802 school attendees; the mean age at first sexual intercourse was 11.4 years. Only 38% were monogamous and only 23% reported consistent use of condoms during sexual intercourse. Twenty percent had a previous homosexual activity and 20% reported intercourse with a partner who injected drugs. In a study of 60 attendees at an inner-city community mental health center in Wisconsin, Kelly and colleagues (1992) noted that 62% of patients had been sexually active in the previous year. Forty-two percent of males and 19% of females had multiple partners. Another Canadian study of 151 outpatients (Chuang and Atkinson, 1996) recorded that 33% of patients had been sexually active in the past month and 52% in the past year. Seventeen percent had sex with more than one partner. Sixteen percent reported sex with a new acquaintance whom they had known less than 24 hours. In a study of homeless men (84% of whom had a psychotic disorder) in a New York City shelter, 53% experienced intercourse in the preceding six months; 31% engaged in homosexual intercourse and 17% of men had bisexual experiences (Susser et al., 1995). Coverdale and colleagues (1997) recently reported on a controlled study in New Zealand of sexual activity among 66 outpatients (54% with a diagnosis of schizophrenia or schizoaffective disorder) and medical clinic attendees, matched for gender and socioeconomic status. Thirty-five patients reported heterosexual intercourse during the past year; another three patients were exclusively homosexual. Thirty-four percent of patients (compared with eight percent of controls) had sex under coercion.

Sexuality in Hospitalized Patients

In the face of liability concerns and a strong prohibition of sexual behavior in hospitals, there is a dearth of information on the sexual activity of inpatients. Systematic research in this contentious area is avoided (Binder, 1985; Chase, 1988; Holbrook, 1989). Mossman and colleagues (1997) provide an excellent account of both scholarly, legal and anectdotal evidence of sex among inpatients. Earlier studies (Akhtar et al., 1977; Modestin, 1981) reported a suspiciously low rate of sexual activity among inpatients. Lyketos and colleagues (1983) examined the sexual behavior of 113 long-stay residents in a Greek psychiatric hospital, and reported a frequency of intercourse of once or twice a month in these patients. More severe psychopathology and longer duration of hospitalization were associated with less sexual activity. The authors concluded that the patient did not "disturb" the social millieu of the hospital or pose a risk to the neighboring community. Anecdotal evidence of sexual behavior among inpatients can also be gleaned from several studies of hospital staff attitudes (Cohen and Tanenbaum, 1985; Welch et al., 1991; Civic et al., 1993). These reports, while convincing and consistent with clinical experience, are more impressionistic in account. In a study of staff attitudes at a 1,000-bed state psychiatric hospital (Civic et al., 1993) sexual contact between patients occurred mostly on hospital grounds. Masturbation in private was allowed on the units. Sexual activity of varied expression was common. Staff expressed real concern regarding sexual bartering and victimization of vulnerable patients; no details were given on the actual extent and pattern of sexual behavior in this hospital. Similarly, Cohen and Tanenbaum (1985) confirmed the occurrence of sex among inpatients but no details of incidents or sexual activity are provided. Holbrook (1989) acknowledged the fear and potential adverse consequences of reporting such data in state hospitals.

Thus, in contrast to an extensive literature on sex in the community setting, the true extent of sexual expression among inpatients is unknown. To address this issue, we recently examined the extent of inpatient sexual behavior as recorded by 57 state hospital administrators (Buckley and Hyde, 1997). Twenty-six percent considered sexual behavior to be a persistent concern in their institution.

Patterns of Sexual Behavior

Sexual activity may represent normal sexual expression or may be related to psychotic symptoms, institutional subculture, or any combination thereof. Patterns of sexual practices among persons with serious mental illness are detailed in Tables 1.3 and 1.4. In general terms, the literature supports the viewpoint that sexual activity is more likely to reflect *normal* sexual desire and expression than to be illness-related. This is an important point to emphasize (also see Deegan, this book). Similarly, the pattern of high-risk behaviors – i.e., unprotected sex, sex with drug-abusing partners – broadly parallels the pattern in the general population. However, since this is a population at-risk for HIV infection (Grassi 1996; also see McKinnon and Cournos, this volume) knowledge of the practices and risk behaviors of patients is important and should be a part of the comprehensive psychiatric evaluation.

Some commentary on particular behaviors is warranted. Reports of rates of homosexual experiences (see Table 1.4) are higher than in the general population (see earlier section). Many patients have social skills deficits and may socialize easier with other patients of the same sex. Hospitalization in single sex wards may reinforce this. Rates of masturbation among the seriously mentally ill are high. Rozensky and Berman (1984) reported that 89% of patients engaged in masturbation. Forty-five percent of patients reported masturbatory activity at a frequency of two or more times a week. This may be the only form of sexual expression. Public masturbation for many patients is particularly problematic and a reason for frequent rehospitalization and or jail incarceration.

Exchanging sex for money or others goods is another worrisome practice. Deficits intrinsic to the illness, active psychotic symptoms, cognitive impairments and the institutional subculture collectively increase the vulnerability of patients to exploitative sexual relationships. Kelly and colleagues (1992) noted that 13% of outpatients reported sex in exchange for money, drugs, or shelter. In their subsequent study (Kalichman *et al.*, 1994), 43% of patients were coerced to engage in sex. Eighteen percent had received payment for sex. In another community sample, 50% of patients had exchanged sex for money or goods (Cournos *et al.*, 1994); this behavior was equally distributed between male and female patients. Sex exchange behavior was associated with more promiscuous sexual relations. Some commentaries have suggested that sex exchange behavior may be a particularly strong incentive for sexual activity among inpatients (Civic *et al.*, 1993). However, specific data to support this notion are presently lacking.

The Northcoast Study

We have recently examined the sexual practices of inpatients with schizophrenia treated at a state facility. The South Campus hospital of Northcoast Behavioral Healthcare System is a 240-bed hospital providing long-term rehabilitative care. Seventy percent of patients have a diagnosis of schizophrenia. The hospital has a well-formulated policy that explicitly prohibits sexual relationships between patients. However, as with other similar facilities throughout the country (Buckley and Hyde, 1997), informal staff observations indicated that some patients were sexually active. In an effort to quantify and detail the extent and pattern of sexual behavior (with a view to implementing an appropriate psychosexual program) we undertook a formal study of sexuality among these inpatients. The SERBAS, an established scale that has been extensively used to examine sexual behavior in psychiatric patients (McKinnon et al., 1993), was obtained from the authors and was modified to be applicable for interviewing patients with severe psychosis in our hospital. The final 45-item questionnaire was administered to 190 inpatients by a trained research assistant (another assistant completed the first 15 interviews). The questionnaire included details on early childhood experiences, attitudes to sexuality, sexual preferences and behavior patterns. Sexual activity was defined as vaginal intercourse.

Patients who resided on specialized units for mental retardation, psychogeriatrics, or those who were physically impaired were not approached for interview. Sixty-three patients declined or were unable to participate in the study; a minority of these patients either failed to complete the interview or gave answers that were incomprehensible and clearly invalid data. Of the remaining 127 patients, 41 reported that they had been sexually active (i.e., had sexual intercourse) during the preceding six months. The mean age of this patient group was 40 ± 8 years. They had a mean of 8 ± 9 previous hospitalizations in the state mental health system and the duration of their current hospitalization was 6 ± 7 years. Thirty-one had a diagnosis of schizophrenia and 6 had a diagnosis of schizoaffective disorder; the remainder had primary affective disorder or other disorders. Their pattern of sexual behavior is summarized in Table 1.5. Surprisingly, just under 1/2 of these patients reported being in a formal (often longstanding, stable) relationship, i.e., 70% of those in relationships retained partners for over 1 year. Sexual activity took place in multiple locations, with limited privacy. Approximately half of the patients used condoms during intercourse; despite the availability of condoms (upon request) from hospital staff. Less than 1/3 of patients reported frequent use of adequate contraception.

These findings confirm the informal, but nevertheless almost universal, impression of sexual activity among some patients with schizophrenia who reside long-term in state facilities. While these preliminary results are provocative, providing actual data and figures rather than impressionistic accounts, there are several important methodological concerns that must be borne in mind when interpreting these data. It is important to emphasize that these results refer to only a subsample (67%) of patients who were initially approached

Table 1.5. Pattern of Sexual Behavior Among 41 Patients.

In a formal relationship	49%
Length of relationship	
less than 1 year	30%
1–5 years	50%
6+ years	20%
Public masturbation	22%
Sexual abuse as a child	27%
Location of sexual activity	
In bedroom	22%
On hospital grounds	7%
Multiple locations	63%
Undecided/no comment	8%
Types of birth control methods	
Withdrawal	2%
Condoms	49%
Contraceptive pill	2%
None	37%
Other/undecided	10%
Frequency of birth control method use	
Always/frequent	29%
Infrequent/never	39%
Undecided/no comment	32%

regarding this study. Accordingly, it is plausible that more patients may be sexually active than is disclosed by this study. Some patients may have been intimidated by the study and declined to participate. Similarly, of those who did participate, some may have chosen to deny any sexual activity, perceiving that the confidential nature of the interview would not be upheld and that information might be passed on to the patient's treatment team. All participants signed an informed consent form which explicitly stated that this was a confidential interview. Also, the research assistant re-emphasized this point at the onset of the interview. Nevertheless, the potential impact of fear of a breach of confidentiality cannot be underestimated and must be considered as a serious potential confound of these data; particularly at a long-stay facility where confidentiality and personal privacy is at a premium (Chase, 1988). Additionally, many of the patients carried a forensic status and they may have purposefully minimized their sexual activity so that their forensic privilege status would not be jeopardized. At a more fundamental level, patients may have felt intruded upon by this study, particularly by the inevitably intimate nature of many of the questions. This certainly could have influenced the pattern of responses. Finally, these patients had severe psychosis and their response to questions may have been impaired by either positive symptoms (especially paranoid) and/or cognitive dysfunction. McEvoy has reported similar difficulties when interviewing patients about explicit sexual details (McEvoy et al., 1983). Patients with primary mental retardation or dementia were excluded from the study, as were those who completed or partially completed interviews in which answers were clearly incorrect. The SERBAS scale which was modified (and shortened) for use in this study was designed for interviewing of psychiatric patients. Its reliability and validity testing are reported elsewhere as acceptable (Meyer-Bahlburg et al., 1990). However, the population in our state hospital had severe illness and they may perhaps be more susceptible than other patient groups to give inappropriate answers to questions. In instances where we considered this to have occurred (such as the number of sexual partners) a conservative approach was taken to interpreting the data. In the study by Lyketsos and colleagues (1983), severe psychopathology was associated with less sexual activity. Patients with severe illness may have been less sexually active. Alternatively, they may have been less forthcoming when interviewed because of the severity of their severity of their psychosis. Cournos and colleagues (1994) have reported the opposite; namely, that sexual activity is associated with more prominent psychopathology. However, this latter study was based upon a community sample as opposed to a long-stay hospital population. We did not conduct a formal cognitive assessment of patients who participated in this study; the study design would have been improved by the inclusion of some brief test of cognitive function such as the mini mental status test. It should be emphasized that these design issues are not trivial points in conducting research in this area. We highlight these to sensitize others who may plan similar research. These points are also relevant when considering the best approach to the assessment of sexual behavior (see earlier).

Notwithstanding these important limitations, some observations may be made from this preliminary analysis. Less than 1/3 of patients who were sexually active recorded that their behavior was confined to the privacy of a bedroom. Sixty-three percent reported having sex in multiple locations on the hospital grounds. In accordance with the studies conducted in community samples (Kelly et al., 1992; Cournos et al., 1994; Grassi, 1996), most patients did not consistently use birth control methods, even though condoms were available upon request. This suggests that patients may be exposed to the risk of STDs in spite of apparently adequate safeguards by the institution.

Sexual Activity and Other Psychiatric Disorders

Sexual activity may be increased or decreased in other psychiatric disorders. For example, anorexia nervosa is typically associated with hyposexuality and fears of sexuality, especially in males (Buckley *et al.*, 1991). Sexual interest and activity may vary greatly with mood. Depression is typically associated with decreased sexual interest, libido and sexual performance (Bhui and Puffett, 1994). Moreover, most of the commonly used antidepressant medications impair sexual functioning and compound the lack of sexual desire during episodes of depression (see Chapter 10). On the other hand, mania is associated with disinhibition, impulsivity and overfamiliarity. Manic patients may engage in high-risk behaviors and show disinhibition with promiscuity. Some studies have compared sexual activity between patients with schizophrenia and mood disorders. Volavka and colleagues reported that HIV seropositivity was higher in females with bipolar disorder than in schizophrenia or other diagnoses (Volavka *et al.*, 1991). In a recent study, Chuang and Atkinson (1996) reported no difference in patterns of sexual behavior between patients with schizophrenia (n = 69), bipolar disorder (n = 37), or unipolar depression (n = 35). Susser and colleagues (1995) reported that homeless men with non-psychotic diagnoses were more likely than those who were psychotic to have multiple partners and to engage in unprotected intercourse. Cournos and colleagues (1993) reported similar rates of sexual activity (53%) between patients with schizophrenia and patients with affective disorder.

Patients with personality disorders may have disturbed sexual relationships. For example, instability of interpersonal relationships is a diagnostic criterion for borderline personality disorder (BPD). In a study of sexual practices among 80 patients with BPD, Zubenko and colleagues (1987) reported that 53% of males and 11% of females were homosexual in orientation. Five percent of patients were bisexual in orientation and 11% had comorbid diagnoses of paraphilias. In contrast, sexual interest is diminished in other personality disorders, such as schizoid, schizotypal or paranoid personality disorders. The latter type are prone to suspicions of sexual infidelity and may develop morbid jealousy or erotomania that is associated with a significant risk of aggression towards the partner.

The sexual behaviors of individuals with mental retardation have been the subject of particular scrutiny (Bhui and Puffett, 1994). It has been suggested that sexual offenses and paraphilias are more common among this group. Additionally, this population are particularly vulnerable to sexual abuse, either from staff or from other individuals with mental retardation. Consequently, the issues of competency, conceptive control, and litigation have received much attention in this patient group (Bhui and Puffett, 1994).

Alcoholism is traditionally associated with heightened sexual activity, predominately due to the social contact and disinhibition associated with chronic alcohol use (Stall *et al.*, 1986). However, sexual performance is impaired with increasing alcohol use. Prolonged alcohol abusers are prone to reduced libido, anorgasmia, erectile dysfunction and ejaculatory difficulties. These may result from the direct intoxication effects of alcohol or may emerge as a part of an alcohol-related neuropathy and endocrine failure.

Sexual activity in persons suffering with mental illness is particularly likely when they also abuse alcohol or drugs (Kelly *et al.*, 1992; Silberstein and Galanter, 1994). In a study of 60 patients, of whom 62% had been sexually active in the previous year, 55% reported alcohol used, 15%, marijuana used, 18% cocaine use, and 5% had injected illicit drugs in the past year (Kelly *et al.*, 1992). Patients gave histories of trading sex for drugs or sexual activity that was directly related to substance use. Silberstein and Galanter (1994) reported that 23% of persons with dual diagnosis (substance abuse and primary psychiatric disorder) admitted to an inpatient unit were HIV positive.

CONCLUSION

It is evident that many patients with severe mental illness have active and fulfilling sexual lives. This contrasts with the apparently smaller number of patients whose sexual behavior is inappropriate and predatory. The actions of the latter group have overshadowed the needs of the majority of persons with mental illness and have had greater impact on public policy in this realm. The whole aspect of patient exploitation and victimization is largely unexplored and is fertile for substantial research. Moreover, this would generate data to inform clinicians so that they could better address the wider issue of normal sexuality among persons with mental illness.

REFERENCES

Abernathy, V. (1974). Sexual knowledge, attitudes, and practices of young female psychiatry patients. *Arch Gen Psychiatry* 30:180–182.

ACSF investigators (1992). Aids and sexual behaviour in France. *Nature* 360: 407–409.

Akhtar, S., Crocker, E., Dickey, N. *et al.* (1977). Overt sexual behavior among psychiatric inpatients. *Diseases of the Nervous System* 38:359–361.

Akhtar, S. and Thompson, J.A. (1980). Schizophrenia and sexuality: a review and a report of twelve unusual cases–part I. *Journal of Clinical Psychiatry* 41(4):134–142.

Akhtar, S. & Thompson, J.A. (1980). Schizophrenia and sexuality: a review and a report of twelve unusual cases–part II. *Journal of Clinical Psychiatry* 41(5):166–174.

Baker, D.G. & Mossman, D. (1991). Potential HIV exposure in psychiatrically ill hospitalized adolescent girls. *American Journal of Psychiatry* 148:528–530.

Bhui, K. & Puffel, A. (1994). Sexual problems in the psychiatric and mentally handicapped populations. *British Journal of Hospital Medicine* 51(9):459–464.

Binder, R.L. (1985). Sex between psychiatric patients. *Psychiatric Quarterly* 57(2):12–126.

Buckley, P.F., Freyne, A. & Walsh, N. (1991). Anorexia nervosa in males. *Irish Journal of Psychological Medicine* 8:15–18.

Buckley, P.F. & Hyde, J.L. (1997). State hospital's responses to the sexual behavior of psychiatric inpatients. *Psychiatric Services* 48:398–399.

Burke, M.A., McEvoy, J.P. & Ritchie, J.C. (1994). A pilot study of a structured interview addressing sexual function in men with schizophrenia. *Biological Psychiatry* 35:32–35.

Chase, J.C. (1988). Sexual drive of patients in psychiatric hospitals. *British Medical Journal* 297:1129.

Chuang, H.T. & Atkinson, M. (1996). AIDS knowledge and high-risk behaviour in the chronic mentally ill. *Canadian Journal of Psychiatry* 41: 269–272.

Civic, D., Walsh, G. & McBride, D. (1993). Staff perspectives on sexual behavior of patients in a state psychiatric hospital. *Hospital and Community Psychiatry* 44(9):887–889.

Cohen, D.D. & Tanenbaum, R.L. (1985). Sexuality education for staff in long-term psychiatric hospitals. *Hospital and Community Psychiatry* 36(2): 187–189.

Cournos, F., Empfield, M., Horwarth, E., McKinnon, K. *et al.* (1991). HIV seroprevalence among patients admitted to two psychiatric hospitals. *American Journal of Psychiatry* 148:1225–1230.

Cournos, F., Guido, J.R., Coomaraswamy, S. *et al.* (1994). Sexual activity and risk of HIV infection among patients with schizophrenia. *American Journal of Psychiatry* 151(2):228–232.

Cournos, F., McKinnon, K., Meyer-Bahlburg, H. *et al.* (1993). HIV risk activity among persons with severe mental illness: preliminary findings. *Hospital and Community Psychiatry* 44:1104–1106.

Coverdale, J.H., Turbott, S.H. & Roberts, H. (1997). Family planning needs and STD risk behaviors of female psychiatric outpatients. *British Journal of Psychiatry* 171:69–72.

Coverdale, J.H., Bayer, T.L., McCullough, L.B. & Chervenak, F.A. (1993). Respecting the autonomy of chronic mentally ill women in decisions about contraception. *Hospital and Community Psychiatry* 44(7):671–674.

Crawford, M.J. & Shaw, T. (1998). Psychiatric outpatients views on talking about sex. *Psychiatric Bulletin* 22:365–367.

Diclemente, R.J. & Ponton, L.E. (1993). HIV-related risk behaviors among psychiatrically hospitalized adolescents and school-based adolescents. *American Journal of Psychiatry* 150:324–325.

Friedman, S. & Harrison, G. (1984). Sexual histories, attitudes and behavior of schizophrenic and "normal" women. *Archives of Sexual Behavior* 13(6):555–567.

Grassi, L. (1996). Risk of HIV infection in psychiatrically ill patients. *AIDS CARE* 8(1):103–116.

Holbrook, T. (1989). Policing sexuality in a modern state hospital. *Hospital and Community Psychiatry* 40(1):75–79.

Johnson, A.M., Wadsworth, J., Wellings, K. *et al.* (1992). Sexual lifestyles and HIV risk. *Nature* 360:410–412.

Kalichman, S.C., Kelly, J.A., Johnson, J.R. & Buero, M. (1994). Factors associated with risk for HIV infection among chronic mentally ill adults. *American Journal of Psychiatry* 151:221–227.

Katz, R.C., Watts, C. & Santman, J. (1994). AIDS knowledge and high risk behaviors in the chronic mentally ill. *Community Mental Health Journal* 30:395–402.

Keefe, R.S.E., Mohs, R.C., Losonczy, M.F., Davidson, M., Silverman, J.M., Horvath, T.B. & Davis, K.L. (1989). Premorbid sociosexual functioning and long-term outcome in schizophrenia. *American Journal of Psychiatry* 146(2):206–211.

Keitner, G. & Grof, P. (1981). Sexual and emotional intimacy between psychiatric inpatients: Formulating a policy. *Hospital and Community Psychiatry* 32(3):188–193.

Kelley, M.E., Gilbertson, M., Mouton, A. *et al.* (1992). Deterioration in premorbid functioning in schizophrenia: a developmental model of negative symptoms in drug-free patients. *American Journal of Psychiatry* 149:1543–1548.

Kelly, J.A., Murphy, D.A., Bahr, G.R., Brasfield, T.L., Davis, D.R. & Hauth, H.C. (1992). AIDS/HIV risk behavior among the chronic mentally ill. *American Journal of Psychiatry* 149:886–889.

Lukoff, D., Sullivan, J.G. & Goisman, R.M. (1992). Sex and AIDS education. (Eds. Liberman, R.P., Goldstein, A.P. and Krasner, L.) Allyn and Bacon, Boston, 171–182.

Lyketsos, G.C., Sakka, D. & Mailis, A. (1983). The sexual adjustment of chronic schizophrenics: a preliminary study. *British of Journal Psychiatry* 143: 376–382.

McDermott, B.E., Sautter, F.J., Winstead, D.K. & Quirk, T. (1994). Diagnosis, health beliefs, and risk of HIV infection in psychiatric patients. *Hospital and Community Psychiatry* 45(6):580–585.

McKinnon, K., Cournos, F., Meyer-Bahlburg, H.F.L., Guido, J., Caraballo, L.R., Margoshes, E.S., Herman, R., Gruen, R.S. & Exner, T.M. (1993). Reliability of sexual risk behavior interviews with psychiatric patients. *American Journal of Psychiatry* 150(6):972–974.

Menon, A.S. & Pomerantz, S. (1997). Substance abuse during sex and unsafe sexual behaviors among acute psychiatric inpatients. *Psychiatric Services* 48:1070–1072.

Modestin, J. (1981). Patterns of overt sexual interaction among acute psychiatric inpatients. *Acta Psychiatiatrica Scandinavica* 64:446–459.

Nesteros, J.N., Lehmann, H.E. & Ban, T.A. (1981). Sexual behavior of the male schizophrenic: the impact of illness and medications. *Archives of Sexual Behavior* Vol. 10(5):421–442.

Pinderhughes, C.A., Grace, B.B. & Reyna, L.W. (1972). Psychiatric disorders and sexual functioning. *American Journal of Psychiatry* 128:1276–1283.

Raboch, J. (1986). Sexual development and life of psychiatric female patients. *Archives of Sexual Behavior* 15(4):341–353.

Rozensky, R.H. & Berman, C. (1984). Sexual knowledge, attitudes, and experiences of chronic psychiatric patients. *Psychosocial Rehabilitation Journal* 8(1):21–27.

Seidman, S.N. & Rieder, R.O. (1994). A review of sexual behavior in the United States. *American Journal of Psychiatry* 151(3):330–334.

Shaul, S. & Morrey, L. (1980). Sexuality education in a state mental hospital. *Hospital and Community Psychiatry* 31(3):175–179.

Silberstein, C., Galanter, M., Marmor, M. *et al.* (1994). HIV-1 among inner city dually diagnosed inpatients. *American Journal of Drug and Alcohol Abuse* 20:201–213.

Stall, R., McKusick, L., Wiley, J., Coates, T.J. & Ostrow, D.G. (1986). Alcohol and drug use during sexual activity and compliance with safe sex guidelines for AIDS: the AIDS behavioral research project. *Health Education Quarterly* 13(4):359–371.

Susser, E., Valencia, E., Miller, M., Tsai, W.Y. *et al.* (1995). Sexual behaviour of homeless mentally ill men at risk for HIV. *American Journal of Psychiatry* 152:583–587.

Vandereycken, W. (1993). Shrinking sexuality: The half-known sex life of psychiatric patients. *Therapeutic Communities* 14(3):143–149.

Volvaka, J., Convit, A., Czobor, P., Douyon, R., O'Donnell, J. & Ventura, F. (1991). HIV seroprevalence and risk behaviors in psychiatric inpatients. *Psychiatry Research* 39:109–114.

Volvaka, J., Convit, A., Czobor, P., Douyon, R., O'Donnell, J. & Ventura, F. (1992). Assessment of risk behaviours for HIV infection among psychiatric inpatients. *Hospital and Community Psychiatry* 43:482–485.

Welch, S., Meagher, J., Soos, J. & Bhopal, J. (1991). Sexual behavior of hospitalized chronic psychiatric patients. *Hospital and Community Psychiatry* 42(8):855–856.

Zubenko, G.S., Anselm, W.G., Soloff, P.H. & Schulz, P. (1987). Sexual practices among patients with borderline personality disorder. *American Journal of Psychiatry* 144:748–752.

2

Human Sexuality and Mental Illness: Consumer Viewpoints and Recovery Principles

PATRICIA E. DEEGAN

Those of us who have been diagnosed with major mental illness do not cease to be human beings by virtue of that diagnosis. Like all people we experience the need for love, companionship, solitude, and intimacy. Like all people we want to feel loved, valued, and desired by others.

The greatest and most healing service that can be offered to people with psychiatric disabilities is to treat them with respect and honor them as human beings. This means honoring us in our full humanity, including our sexuality and our desire to love and be loved.

In the spirit of honoring the full humanity of people diagnosed with major mental illness, I invited a group of people to discuss how mental health services affect our sexuality and our capacity to love. All of the members of the group were diagnosed with major mental illness, have had multiple hospitalizations, and are receiving a wide range of mental health services including residential and case management. I found the stories and insights shared in our discussion to be inspirational and filled with humor, common sense and wisdom. They deserve thoughtful reflection, and so I have organized this paper around the themes which emerged in that discussion. These themes include:

- Psychiatric medications and sexuality
- The reduction of sexuality to psychopathology

- The need for clear and comprehensive policies regarding sex and romance in mental institutions
- The possibility that mental institutions (and not the sexuality of the people in them) are problematic
- The unnecessary practices that shame and humiliate us

In addition to reflecting on the group's comments, I will also outline principles of the recovery model that can inform and guide decision-making regarding human sexuality and mental illness.

Psychiatric Medications and Sexuality

My biggest problem with sex is medication. These pharmaceutical companies should warn you and they don't. They don't warn us about the sexual side effects. The pharmaceutical companies should put the warning right on the bottle.

All members of the focus group echoed the theme expressed by this first speaker. We all felt psychiatric medications had interfered with our sexual function and/or desire. For some, the problem with medications was ongoing. For others, it had been resolved either by going off the medication or changing it.

This first speaker suggests a warning be placed directly on the pill bottle. He clearly would have preferred to know about possible drug effects on his sexuality before he took it. I would add that it is also his legal right to be informed directly about drug effects by the prescribing physician or nurse practitioner. Thorough discussions of unwanted drug effects, however, were not the norm in our group's experience. Rather, many of us had never been informed about possible sexual dysfunction related to medication use or concomitant emotional blunting, anhedonia, apathy, indifference, anorgasmia, and reduction in sex drive. We tended to blame ourselves for our sexual dysfunction and subsequently felt ashamed and fearful of engaging in intimate relationships. Most of us learned about these medication effects from peers who used the drugs or from reading about the drugs in books that we found on our own which were not provided by mental health centers or professionals.

One member of the group said he did report his sexual dysfunction to his psychiatrist: *I have the problem that my medication gives me which is premature ejaculation. They keep telling me, "You have to be on this medication. There is no other medication you can be on. You have to accept this side effect." I don't think I should have to accept this side effect. They want me to commit sexual suicide.*

The option of "sexual suicide" is unacceptable and only sets this speaker up for eventual medication non-compliance. When most of us with psychiatric disabilities encounter drug effects that impair our quality of life, we want to be able to work collaboratively with our doctors/nurse practitioners to find alternatives. Remember that alternatives include other medications, different dosages, as well as the opportunity to learn non-drug coping strategies to eliminate or decrease distressing symptoms (Deegan, 1995).

Never tell people they will have to stay on medications for the rest of their lives. Such a message is utterly demoralizing and empirically unfounded (Harding & Zahniser, 1994). Rather, always suggest a trial period. Put a reasonable time frame around the length of the drug trial. Most people can endure uncomfortable or disabling drug effects if there is a firm rationale for expecting a good outcome from the drug trial and if they know there is an end point at which the outcome of the trial will be collaboratively discussed.

When evaluating a person's long-term medication use, take the time to inquire about unwanted effects. Some people have become so accustomed to sexual dysfunction and/or loss of sexual desire they may not even mention it. In taking the time to reach out to these people and explore medication reductions, changing medications and self help strategies, care is demonstrated for the *whole* person and the overall quality of his/her life.

The Reduction of Sexuality to Psychopathology

On the one hand they don't let you have sexual relationships with other people when you're in the hospital. On the other hand they say you can't masturbate. They say the reason you can't masturbate is because of the thoughts you might have later. They say there's nothing wrong with masturbation but that the thoughts it might stir up would cause you problems later in the day.

The association between sexual acts and "problems" is not new. Throughout the history of American psychiatry the sexuality of people diagnosed with mental illness has been suspect. Under the lens of medical/institutional scrutiny, that which was private became open to clinical scrutiny and academic debate. Historically, sexuality has been reduced to either the cause or symptom of psychopathology.

Masturbation has been understood as a primary cause of mental disorders. In the 18th century the father of American psychiatry, Benjamin Rush, wrote a chapter, "Of the Morbid state of the Sexual Appetite." He claimed that onanism (masturbation) "produces seminal weakness, impotence, dysury, tabes dorsalis, pulmonary consumption, dyspepsia, dimness of sight, vertigo, epilepsy, hypochondriasis, loss of memory, manalgia, fatuity, and death." (Rush, 1812, p. 347) A century later Samuel Woodward, the founder of the American Psychiatric Association, echoed Rush's concern about masturbation. Loss of semen was thought to be debilitating and could lead to madness and even death. In an introduction to Sylvester Graham's *A Lecture to Young Men on Chastity* (1839), Woodward wrote "The evil of which [this book] treats . . . is more extensively sapping the foundation of physical vigor and moral purity, in the rising generation, than is generally apprehended even by those who are awake to the danger," (Gamwell & Tomes, 1995, p. 112).

In 1888, the physician John Harvey Kellogg noted the dire effects of masturbation upon the nerves of young men. He wrote, "In the insane asylums of the country may be seen hundreds of these poor victims in all stages of physical and mental demoralization" (Gamwell & Tomes, 1995, p. 112). Although women were also swelling the ranks of mental institutions, physicians and psychiatrists of the 19th and early 20th century did not generally attribute this insanity to indulgence in the 'secret vice'. Rather insanity in women was, in many cases, thought to be caused by a defect or irritation of the reproductive organs, especially the uterus (Geller & Harris, 1994). Treatment included the administration of various vegetable and mineral tonics as well as opiates to calm the excited uterus. Physicians judged that women who appeared excited during menstruation should have their ovaries removed in an effort to calm them. An ovarian restraining apparatus was devised. In an effort to calm the agitated uterine system, physicians injected hot water into a woman's vagina. They developed a procedure to cauterize a woman's clitoris. In women who were not virgins, an apparatus called the double uterine exciter was indicated. It "applied an electrical current to the uterus" and "was employed for periods lasting up to ten minutes." (Geller & Harris, 1994, p. 100–111)

The eugenics movement marked another wave in the assault on the sexuality of people diagnosed with mental illness. In America the eugenics movement was marked by an effort to purify and insure the dominance of the white Anglo Saxon race. One of the methods devised to achieve this end was sterilization or the "asexualization of the unfit" (Barr, 1912, 1915). People considered unfit included convicted rapists and criminals, people with mental retardation and people judged insane. By 1907 Indiana passed the first state laws permitting sterilization. By 1931, thirty states had passed sterilization laws and over 20,000 people had been sterilized (Bell, 1980).

Another reduction of sexuality to a form of psychopathology is illustrated in psychiatry's view of homosexuality. As Gamwell and Tomes (1995, p. 111) summarize, in 1932 the American Medical Association, in conjunction with the American Psychiatric Association, classified homosexuality as a psychopathic personality disorder in the Standard Classified Nomenclature of Disease. In 1952 the American Psychiatric Association included homosexuality as a sociopathic personality disorder in the first Diagnostic and Statistical Manual of Psychiatric Disorders. It wasn't until 1973 that homosexuality was removed from the DSM.

As a person with a psychiatric disability, I feel a combination of outrage, sadness and fear when I read about what has been done to us in the name of treatment. I am horrified that society would seek to protect itself against those of us with mental illness by sanctioning mass violence against us (albeit this violence was in the guise of treatment). Never has a single person or organization of people with mental illness perpetrated violence on such a scale. It has only been normal, non-diagnosed people who have been empowered by our society to treat tens of thousands of mental patients through the use of forced sterilization, clitoral cauterization, applying electrical currents to reproductive organs and incarceration of gay men and lesbians.

I understand mental health professionals' intent is to help people, not to hurt people. However, they must not avert their eyes from the facts of history. The track record regarding the sexuality of people diagnosed with mental illness is not very good. The temptation of dismissing the past as past must be avoided. It will not do to rest comfortably in the illusion that today's clinicians live in a scientific age in which their work is guided solely by empirical progress (Kuhn, 1970). Rather, mental health professionals must learn from the past and dare to question the assumptions which guide their work and the very questions they ask about their work. For instance, they might ask:

- Where are the programs in the service system that provide in-home supports and skills training for parents with major mental illness and their children? Where are the residential programs for married couples or single parents with children? If these services do not exist, what does that say about assumptions regarding the sexuality of people with major mental illness?
- How are inpatient units and community based programs organized to be inclusive of people who are gay, lesbian or bi-sexual? How are gay, lesbian and bi-sexual men and women who also have major mental illness, assisted in coping with the double discrimination they encounter? How are issues of staff homophobia and heterosexism addressed in programs? If these issues are not being addressed, what does this say about assumptions regarding the sexuality of people diagnosed with major mental illness?
- When a woman is using neuroleptics do we consider the abatement of her psychotic symptoms more important than the fact that she also develops amenorrhea and loses her reproductive capacity while on the drug(s)?
- How is a woman with major mental illness who is approaching 40 years of age and states her intent to "have a child before it is too late" counseled? How are genetic studies of the incidence of schizophrenia and affective disorders interpreted? Do clinicians oversimplify and tell clients that mental illnesses are genetically transmitted in a linear, causal, and/or deterministic way? Is the eugenics agenda at work in such consultation?

- Are there services in place to support a pregnant woman in discontinuing her psychiatric medications to ensure the safety of her baby? If these services are not available, what does that say about assumptions regarding the sexuality of people with major mental illness.

The Need for Clear and Comprehensive Policies Regarding Sex and Romance in Mental Institutions

First they tell you there is no sex allowed in the hospital. Then they pass out condoms and tell you to be sure to use them for safe sex.

This member of the focus group captures the mixed messages that are sent to people in mental institutions regarding sexuality and romance. Instructing patients in the No Physical Contact Rule and then supplying condoms is contradictory and confusing both for the staff who are expected to enforce the rule and for the patients who are supposed to abide by it.

Most hospital units have an obligatory policy statement regarding patient sexuality. However, a policy prohibiting sex does not necessarily eliminate it. For instance, in one study looking at the sexual activity of women diagnosed with schizophrenia in a long-term institution, 65% of women reported having intercourse while in the hospital during the prior three months (McEvoy, Hatcher, Appelbaum & Abenethy, 1983). Despite the official policy prohibiting sex, the operational policy in many inpatient settings is something akin to "Don't ask, don't tell; don't look, don't see." A comprehensive policy addressing the real issues is required.

When you're in the hospital you feel the most vulnerable. You are going through a lot of pain and suffering. Reaching out to someone is healing and reassuring. But then your psychiatrist says that if you reach out for intimacy, love, affection, touch . . . that is about being predatory. That's about taking advantage of vulnerable people. That's inappropriate.

This member of the focus group clearly states the tension he experiences regarding life in an institution, including short term and intermediary stay units. He does not cease to be a human being with needs for intimacy and comfort upon being diagnosed or admitted to a mental institution. In fact, in an institution loneliness and pain can be amplified. In such circumstances it is quite natural for anyone to seek solace in the warmth of an embrace. This group member sees interpersonal physical affection and love as something that could be healing for him. Yet he also reports when he acts on these human needs in an inpatient setting, he is told he is being inappropriate and predatory. He is told the other people in the setting are vulnerable and could be taken advantage of.

A comprehensive policy regarding sexual activity in mental institutions must address the tension so clearly captured in the statement above. A policy must address the needs and the rights of adults to seek intimacy, love, and physical comfort as well as addressing the responsibilities of the institution to protect people from the exploitative and predatory behaviors of both staff and other inpatients. Attorney Susan Stefen (1995, p. 2) suggests a comprehensive policy will:

- Address the prevention of rape and coercive sex
- Contain detailed plans of action in the case of allegation of rape or coercive sex
- Address issues of sex education
- Address issues relating to contraception
- Address issues relating to client pregnancy
- Address issues relating to voluntary sexuality including masturbation and expressions of physical affection short of intercourse
- Address issues of client privacy
- Address HIV/AIDs related issues.

Stefen also suggests mere consent is not a sufficient standard for policies regarding sexuality on inpatient units. She suggests that mutuality and voluntariness are superior standards. "It should not be sufficient to consent: the relationship should be mutually desired by both parties"(Stefen, 1995, p. 5). The standard of mutuality and voluntariness is particularly important in light of the relatively high percentage of men and women with major mental illness who have histories of sexual abuse and who are vulnerable to reenacting that trauma by consenting to unwanted sex.

These issues receive further attention in one chapters by Buckley *et al.* (chap. 4) and by Welch *et al.* (chap. 5).

The Possibility that Mental Institutions (and not the Sexuality of the People in them) are Problematic

I was married for ten years before coming into the hospital. Outsiders never told me what I could and couldn't do sexually in my marriage. And then when I'm in the hospital under their control, the things they are telling me I can't do make me feel like a kid.

This member of the focus group helps us understand that in an institution, what is usually private becomes a matter of public concern. Is it possible to insure privacy for adults who are patients in psychiatric institutions? The very notion of developing a policy that allows privacy and or private space to engage in mutually desired sexual relations in institutions seems aberrant (Stefen, 1995). For instance, how would use of a private room be monitored? Who could use it and who would not be allowed to use such a room? Would the room be available 24 hours a day or just at certain times? Would use of the private room be considered a privilege or a right or a clinical issue? What if a couple ran overtime in the private room? How would they be informed that another couple might be waiting and who would inform them?

As one begins to grapple with the mechanics of a policy that would allow privacy in an institutional setting, it becomes clear it is the institutional setting itself, not the inmates of that institution, which is unnatural and problematic. The problem is not that people diagnosed with major mental illness want to engage in intimate relationships. The problem is that institutions strip away their control over what remains private and what they choose to make public. Perhaps, rather than focusing efforts on controlling the sexual expression of people in mental institutions, time should be spent considering the possibility of dismantling such institutions and working with people in their own homes, in the context of their ongoing lives.

Knowing that the dismantling of mental institutions will be a long time coming, Stefen (1995) suggests a middle ground. She suggests that:

> all institutions should provide on each ward a private room where a client can go to get away from the chaos and overstimulation on the ward. People who have been institutionalized, particularly with histories of sexual abuse, describe repeatedly the crucial and desperate need for a place to be private, alone, and quiet. A client could get a key to this room from a staff member, and could lock herself in and perhaps listen to music on headphones, read, write, draw, or simply be still. If the time came that a decision was made that voluntary and mutual sex was permissible in the case of certain residents, the room would already exist. (p. 7)

The Unnecessary Practices that Shame and Humiliate Us

I kicked over a clothes hamper. I did it on purpose. They tied me in four point restraint for 12 hours plus they shot me up with drugs. I'm not a horse! They left me tied up in just my underwear. There were both men and women staff when I was in restraint. They left the door open. A guard sat in the doorway watching me and people passing in the hall could see me. They treat you like an animal. It's not helpful. I felt ashamed. I lost my appetite. It makes you worse.

This focus group member graphically describes the shame, degradation, and humiliation he experienced while in mechanical and chemical restraint. It is significant that he made this comment in the context of a focus group on sexuality and mental illness. For decades ex-patients have been drawing an analogy between rape and the experience of being forcibly restrained and injected with psychotropic drugs (Chamberlin, 1977; Burstow & Weitz, 1988; Pritchard, 1995). Just as rape and violence can damage human sexuality, so too can restraint. It can be traumatic. Such trauma and wounds to our self esteem linger long after hospitalization. Indeed, it can often be more difficult to recover from these iatrogenic wounds than from mental illness (Deegan, 1990; 1993).

I've been in restraint and seclusion. They keep the cuffs loose. I don't see the reason for it, though. It's supposed to be therapeutic but I can't figure that out.

New Zealand and a number of provinces in Canada have learned to completely eliminate the use of mechanical restraints in mental institutions. An increase in staff to patient ratio has been the key to changing long held attitudes about the need for it. In the United States there is a growing awareness of how mechanical restraints can re-traumatize people with major mental illness who have histories of sexual abuse. For instance the Massachusetts Department of Mental Health Task Force on Restraint and Seclusion of Persons who have been Physically or Sexually Abused (Carmen *et al.*, 1996) has published its recommendations which include: banning forms of physical restraint that require a patient's legs be spread apart; exploring with the patient alternatives to restraint and including these alternatives in the treatment plan; insuring that the staff person assigned to the 1:1 during and after restraint is not the same gender as the patient's sexual abuse perpetrator; and that a Trauma Assessment Form and Restraint Reduction form be used as guides to gathering critical information necessary for humane treatment of patients with sexual abuse histories.

There are many other practices which shame and humiliate and in turn, affect the sexuality of mental health clients. Some of the others that were mentioned in the focus group included procedures for using toilets and showers when on 1:1 as well as wearing johnnies that expose breasts or genitals when on suicide watch. Room checks can interfere with privacy when dressing, especially when staff do not knock. The practice of putting more than one person in a bedroom on inpatient units and in community residential settings is problematic. It interferes with an adult's sexual activity (from masturbation to sexual intimacy with partners). A number of group members complained of lack of privacy during administration of depot injections. Women complain of having to ask male aides or male residential workers for sanitary products. Perhaps the best way to understand the myriad of overt and subtle practices that shame and humiliate people is to organize a focus group of patients/clients who meet to discuss their concerns with administrators on a regular basis. A guide to forming such groups has been developed by Anderson and Deegan (1998).

Recovery Principles

Anthony (1990) declared the 1990's to be the Decade of Recovery. The recovery model recognizes that people can and do recover from major mental illness (Deegan, 1988, 1996; Fisher, 1994) and that the rates of recovery for severe illnesses such as schizophrenia are higher than previously thought (DeSisto, Harding, McCormack, Ashikaga & Gautum, 1995a,b; Harding & Zahniser, 1995). The recovery model emphasizes the person-in-relation – to illness, self, others, social role, society etc. Recovery approaches emphasize the principles of choice, self determination, skill building, self-help, recovery of social role, peer support, and empowerment. The model offers valuable guidelines for working with issues related to human sexuality and mental illness.

One of the fundamental principles of a recovery model is the dignity of risk and the right to failure. This principle was first described by people with physical disabilities (DeJong, 1979) and has been adapted by people with psychiatric disabilities (Deegan, 1992). It is based on the observation that there is a dual standard for people who are diagnosed and those who are not. People who are *not* diagnosed with a major mental illness have the "right" to make self-defeating choices without intervention from authorities wishing to protect them from the consequences of their poor choices. This is best illustrated by thinking of non-diagnosed friends or acquaintances. These people may make poor, uninsightful, self-defeating and even self-endangering choices about sexual partners, marrying again after several divorces, engaging in unprotected sex, being a poor parent yet deciding to have another child, etc. Authorities do not intervene and stop these people from making unwise choices. In other words society accepts that poor judgement and lack of insight are parts of everyday living and that non-diagnosed people can and do make self-defeating choices. Hopefully they learn and grow through such risks and failures. However, once diagnosed with a major mental illness it is often assumed that our behavior is solely determined by the illness. Thus if we make the very same uninsightful or self defeating choices that a non-diagnosed person makes, authorities feel compelled to paternalistic interventions into our lives.

A recovery model recognizes this double standard and urges clinicians and policy makers to distinguish between poor choices and psychopathology. I have worked closely with mental health providers in developing policies regarding consumer choice. In my experience it is helpful to create policy guidelines across the following domains:

- The Comfort Zone: When consumers make choices that providers agree with
- The Conflicted Zone: When consumers make choices that appear to be self defeating or that diminish quality of life
- The Risk Management Zone: When consumer choice becomes a safety and/or liability issue for providers

These domains can be adapted for use in the area of consumer choice and sexuality. Using these domains will help policy makers steer clear of the dual standard described above. It will promote recovery by minimizing paternalism and allowing people the dignity of risk and the right to learn and grow through failure as well as success.

Another principle of the recovery model is to minimize the loss of valued social roles and provide support in the acquisition of new roles after being diagnosed with mental illness. Too often diagnosis with a major mental illness is accompanied by the loss of valued social roles (Fisher, 1998). The loss of roles such as mother, father, worker, community leader, pastor, artist, etc., and the prescription of the role of "persistently mentally ill" has dire consequences for the individual looking to recover from mental illness.

With regard to human sexuality it is imperative that clinicians help clients keep the valued social roles they already have – as lover, spouse, parent or grandparent. Although some clinicians view these roles as possible stressors, they can also be a powerful motivating force for recovery. Lewis (1998, p. 4) reports that one mother in her focus group stated, "Being a mom helped me start thinking as a person instead of as a patient." Mothering has been shown to be a powerful role around which women can re-organize their lives (Mowbray, Oyserman & Ross, 1994; Schwab, Clark & Drake, 1991). In addition, psycho-education for family members and friends regarding the importance of maintaining social roles is helpful. Finally, if functioning in a valued social role is disrupted during the course of the illness, role recovery becomes an important focus of rehabilitation and self-directed recovery.

Another principle of the recovery model is that people can learn non-drug strategies for coping with distressing symptoms. For instance non-drug coping strategies for dealing with major depression (Copeland, 1992), manic depression (Copeland, 1994) and auditory hallucinations (Romme, 1989; Watkins, 1990; Romme & Escher, 1993; Deegan, 1995) have been described. Providing opportunities for people to learn these coping strategies means that many can reduce or completely eliminate the use of psychotropic medications. In turn, medication reduction/discontinuance can lead to the restoration of sexual function.

CONCLUSION

A final principle of the recovery model is to recognize that mental illness is not "all in our head". Mental illness is also a social construct that carries with it all of the stigma and discrimination associated with devalued people. Thus there are many other external, societal factors which affect our sexuality and our capacity to love. For instance mental illness too frequently comes as a package plan that includes poverty, unemployment, poor medical care, marginalization and second-class citizenship. It is difficult to engage in courtship while living below the poverty level on $560 per month. It is difficult to imagine pusuing intimate relationships with people in the community when our neighbors protest the proximity of our group homes. It is difficult to initiate new romantic relationships when the stigma of mental illness is sure to scare most people away. It is difficult to love ourselves when we have internalized the stigma that surrounds us and have learned to hate and fear ourselves.

The problem is not always inside our head. Sometimes the problem of human sexuality and mental illness is found in an unjust society that does not tolerate difference. No amount of medication or psychosocial support is going to cure the dominant culture's discrimination against people with mental illness. Clinicians must be careful not to locate all problems with intimacy and sexuality "inside" of the person with mental illness. We must not fall into the trap of blaming the victim (Ryan, 1976). Sometimes the clinical becomes political and the challenge of striving for a more just society belongs to us all.

REFERENCES

Anderson, D. & Deegan, P.E. (1998). *How to successfully include people with psychiatric disabilities on boards and committees: Overcoming the barriers and providing support* (Available from the National Empowerment Center, 20 Ballard Road, Lawrence MA 01843).

Anthony, W. (1993). Recovery from mental illness: The guiding vision of the mental health service system in the 1990's. *Psychosocial Rehabilitation Journal* 16:11-24.

Barr, M.W. (1912). The asexualization of the unfit. *Alienist and Neurologist* 33:1-9.

Barr, M.W. (1915). The prevention of the mental defect. The duty of the hour. *Alienist and Neurologist* 36:357-364.

Burstow, B. & Weitz, D. (Eds.). (1988). *Shrink resistant: the struggle against psychiatry in Canada*. Vancouver, BC: New Star Books.

Carmen, E., Crane, W., Dunnicliff, M., Holochuck, S., Prescott, L., Rieker, P.P., Stefan, S. & Stromberg, N. (1996). *Massachusetts Department of Mental Health task force on the restraint and seclusion of persons who have been physically or sexually abused : Report and recommendations*. (Available from the Massachusetts Deparment of Mental Health, Central Office 17 Staniford Street, Boston MA 02114).

Chamberlin, J. (1977). *On our own*. United Kingdom: MIND Publications: .

Copeland, M.E. (1992). *The depression workbook: A guide for living with depression and manic depression*. California: New Harbinger Publications, Inc.

Copeland, M.E. (1994). *Living without depression & manic depression: A workbook for maintaining mood stability*. California: New Harbinger Publications, Inc.

Deegan, P.E. (1988). Recovery: The lived experience of rehabilitation. *Psychosocial Rehabilitation Journal* 9, 4:11-19.

Deegan, P.E. (1990). Spirit breaking: When the helping professions hurt. *The Humanistic Psychologist* 18(3):301-313.

Deegan, P.E. (1992). The independent living movement and people with psychiatric disabilities: Taking control back over our own lives. *Psychosocial Rehabilitation Journal* 15:3-19.

Deegan, P.E. (1993). Recovering our sense of value after being labeled mentally ill. *Journal of Psychosocial Nursing* 31(4):7-11.

Deegan, P.E. (1995). *Coping with hearing voices.* (Available from the National Empowerment Center, 20 Ballard Road, Lawrence, MA 01843).

Deegan, P.E. (1996). Recovery as a journey of the heart. *Psychiatric Rehabilitation Journal* 19:91–97.

DeJong, G. (1979). Independent living: From social movement to analytic paradigm. *Archives of Physical Medicine and Rehabilitation* 60:435–446.

DeSisto, M.J., Harding, C.M., McCormick, R.V., Ashikaga, T. & Gautum, S. (1995a). The Maine-Vermont three decades studies of serious mental illness: Matched comparison of cross-sectional outcome. *British Journal of Psychiatry* 167:331–338.

DeSisto, M.J., Harding, C.M., McCormick, R.V., Ashikaga, T. & Gautum, S. (1995b). The Maine-Vermont three decades studies of serious mental illness: Longitudinal course of comparisons. *British Journal of Psychiatry* 167:338–342.

Fisher, D.B. (1994). Health care reform based on an empowerment model of recovery by people with psychiatric disabilities. *Hospital and Community Psychiatry* 45:913–915.

Fisher, D.B. (1998). Recovery: The behavioral healthcare guideline of tomorrow. (Available from the National Empowerment Center, 20 Ballard Road, Lawrence, MA 01843).

Gamwell, L. & Tomes, N. (1995). *Madness in America: Cultural and medical perceptions of mental illness before 1914.* New York : Cornell University Press.

Geller, J.L. & Harris, M. (1994). Women of the asylum. New York: Doubleday.

Harding, C.M. & Zahniser, J.H. (1994). Empirical correction of seven myths about schizophrenia with implications for treatment. *Acta Psychiatrica Scandinavica, 90,* supplement 384:140–146.

Kuhn, T.S. (1970). *The structure of scientific revolutions.* Chicago: University of Chicago Press.

Leland, B.V. (1980). *Treating the mentally ill: From colonial times to the present.* New York: Praeger Publishers.

Lewis, L.R. (1998, April). *A shifting paradigm: Supporting parents with psychiatric disabilities.* Paper presented at the American Orthopsychiatric Association 75th Annual Meeting. (Available through Western Massachusetts Training Consortium, 187 High Street, Holyoke, MA 01040).

McEvoy, J.P., Hatcher, A., Appelbaum, P.S. & Abenethy, V. (1983). Chronic schizophrenic women's attitudes toward sex, pregnancy, birth control, and childrearing. *Hospital and Community Psychiatry* 34(6):536–539.

Mowbray, C.T., Oyserman, D. & Ross, S. (1995). Parenting and the significance of children for women with a serious mental illness. *Journal of Mental Health Administration* 22(2):189–200.

Pritchard, M.(Ed.), (1995). *Dare to vision: Shaping the national agenda for women, abuse and mental health services.* (Available through Human Resource Association of the Northeast, 187 High Street, Holyke, MA 01040).

Romme, M. (1989). Hearing Voices. *Schizophrenia Bulletin* 15(2):209–216.

Romme, M. & Escher, S. (1993). *Accepting Voices.* London, England: MIND Publications, Inc.

Ryan, W. (1976). *Blaming the victim,* New York: Vintage Books.

Rush, B. (1812). *Medical inquiries and observations, upon the diseases of the mind.* Philadelphia.

Schwab, B., Clark, N.E. & Drake, R.E. (1991). An ethnographic note on charts of parents. *Psychosocial Rehabilitation Journal* 15:95–99.

Stefan, S. (1995). Sex in institutional settings: Institutional and agency policies in Massachusetts. *Advisor: Notes From the Mental Health Legal Advisors Committee* 42:1–7.

Watkins, J. (1990). *Hearing voices: A self-help guide and reference book.* Australia: Richmond Fellowship of Victoria.

3

Sex and Mental Illness: Legal Considerations

STEPHEN G. NOFFSINGER

The laws regarding activities related to the sexuality of the mentally ill and mentally retarded face a fundamental tension between the individual's need for (and right to) sexual freedom, and their need for protection from harm (Reed, 1997). On one hand, the mentally ill have an interest in experiencing intimate, caring relationships. This is a critical end often neglected aspect (Deegan, chapter 2). On the other hand, the law must protect those who are vulnerable and unable to give their consent to sexual activities. In addition, disabled persons in the care of the state have a constitutional right to protection from harm.

Sexual activity of mentally ill persons is a controversial topic with a wide range of opinions existing on the topic. On one end of the spectrum patient rights advocates argue that mentally ill individuals have an absolute right to sexual freedom. Patients' Bill of Rights that are an outgrowth of the *Wyatt v. Stickney* (1972) decision often mention mentally ill persons' right to access to the opposite sex for the purpose of fraternization, but usually not sexual encounters. The Therapeutic value of human intimacy is underappreciated (Deegan, chapter 2). At the other end of the spectrum, conservatives argue that the sexual behavior of mentally ill persons must be regulated and that laws governing this area must also factor in general societal interests – that society has an interest in reducing the number of people that are dependent on the state, and since many mental illnesses have a genetic transmission, society has a legitimate interest in this area. Clearly, a broad dichotomy of opinions exists on this often emotionally-charged topic.

The legal aspects of the sexuality of seriously mentally ill persons also involves several discordant issues. Broadly speaking, these issues can be divided into competence to participate in sexual activity and/ or the various activities associated with sex, evaluating sexual assaults in the hospital, and the relationship between legal insanity and serious mental illness, paraphilias and mental retardation.

Competencies Related to Various Sexual Activities

Competence is a broad term that is defined as having the mental ability to understand the nature and effects of one's acts. Over 20 separate types of competence have been identified, varying with regard to the specific act in question. Examples of the various types of competencies include competence to stand trial, competence to be a witness, competence to make a will, and competence to be executed (Gutheil, 1997). Each specific type of competence has a corresponding specific legal definition, determined by statute or case law. (Statutes are laws made by a legislative body, whereas case law is a court's ruling on an issue or interpretation of a law.) For example, competence to stand trial, as determined by the United States Supreme Court in 1960, requires that a defendant have the ability to consult with his lawyer with a reasonable degree of rational understanding, and have a rational as well as factual understanding of the proceedings against him (*Dusky v. United States*, 1960). In comparison, competence to make a will requires that a testator understand the extent of his estate and those who would naturally inherit his possessions.

To further complicate matters, each legal competency may be defined somewhat differently across the statutes or case law of the fifty states or the federal jurisdiction (Grisso, 1986). The standard for competence to manage one's financial affairs may be different in California from the corresponding standard in Idaho, as these standards are often left up to the individual states to determine.

The most frequently encountered competence issues concerning sexual activity among mentally ill persons includes: (1) competence to participate in sexual activity; (2) competence to give informed consent to birth control (pre-intercourse); (3) competence to consent to abortion; (4) competence to parent; and (5) competence to relinquish parental rights. Evaluating the competence of seriously mentally ill patients in these areas is especially important, given that a significant proportion of patients with chronic schizophrenia suffer from defects of cognitive functioning, which could impinge on competence.

Each of the various competencies listed above can be viewed through the perspective of "informed consent." Generally, the law has recognized three factors which must be analyzed in determining whether legally sufficient informed consent for an activity has occurred (Reed, 1997): (1) knowledge of the relevant facts relating to the decision to be made, (2) the intellectual ability to realize and rationally process the risks and benefits of engaging in the proposed activity (i.e., competence); and (3) voluntariness, meaning that the person is not subjected to coercion and that there is a choice between engaging and refraining from the activity. Unfortunately, there has been little elaboration in legal decisions about what constitutes competent decisionmaking. In many jurisdictions the law provides circular definitions: a patient is competent if she is able to give informed consent (Jones, 1995), and able to give informed consent only if competent.

Hospitals have a duty to take reasonable care to protect their patients from the possible harm arising from sexual encounters, and to provide education and rehabilitation relevant to patient sexuality (Welch & Clements, 1996). The hospital administration's duty to protect arises from several sources. In a general sense, the *parens patriae* power of the state carries with it a duty to protect. Moreover, the common law imposes on health care professionals and hospitals a duty to act reasonably and prudently while providing care to patients. The duty to provide education and rehabilitation pertaining to patient sexuality is required as one part of a reasonable effort to protect patients from harm.

This section will address the various competencies relating to sexual activity, the appropriate competency standard, and a method to evaluate competency.

Competency to Participate in Sexual Activity

There are three basic categories of non-consensual sexual intercourse that can be considered a criminal offense: (1) when a person has sex using force or threat of force; (2) when a person is not mentally competent to consent; and (3) when a person is a minor, as defined by state law – also known as statutory rape (Reed, 1997). In regards to incompetence, most states recognize sexual intercourse with a person who does not have the "mental capacity" to consent as a criminal offense. However, as opposed to statutory rape, (where the age of the minor is proof of incompetence) the incompetence of the mentally ill person must be proven. There is a presumption of competence, and the defendant can only be convicted if the mentally ill person has been proven incompetent (lacking "mental capacity") to participate in sexual activity at the time of the sex act.

In Virginia, for example, (Reed, 1997) the state must prove beyond a reasonable doubt that sexual intercourse occurred, that the victim was "mentally incapacitated" at the time of the offense, and that the defendant(s) knew or should have known of the victim's condition. The Texas standard states a man cannot legally have intercourse with a woman if he knows she has "a mental defect to such extent that she is incapable either of appraising the nature of the act of sexual intercourse, or of resisting it." Courts, however, have not provided much guidance on what competence to consent to sexual intercourse specifically means and how the courts should determine whether a person has the mental capacity to consent. Existing standards, while few in number, are controversial. For example, can an incompetent mentally ill man be guilty of rape and subjected to imprisonment if he has consensual intercourse with a peer who is equally incompetent?

Reed (1997) reports that the majority of states interpret "mental incapacity" to mean that the person could not understand the nature of sexual conduct – that is, the person does not know either the physiological aspects of sex, or the possible consequences of sexual activity, such as pregnancy and the contraction of sexually transmitted diseases, including AIDS. A handful of states, most notably New York, have interpreted mental impairment to have a broader meaning. In addition to understanding the nature of the sexual act involved and its consequences, the person must also appreciate the moral dimensions of the decision to engage in sexual conduct, although the individual is free to act inconsistently with these notions of morality. Finally, New Jersey seems to have established the most limited interpretation, requiring an understanding of the sexual and voluntary nature of the act, but not of the risks and consequences of sexual conduct.

Clinical assessment of a mentally ill persons' capacity to engage in sexual activity can be difficult, as few standardized assessment tools exist, of which none has been generally accepted (see Figure 3.1) However, specific items that evaluators should investigate include:

1. The patient's understanding of the nature and consequences of sexual activity. Does the patient understand that their actions

---

1. Socio-Sexual Knowledge and Attitudes Test (SSKAT) (Neiderbuhl and Morris, 1993). The SSKAT includes questions regarding both knowledge and attitudes about sexuality – the questions do not rely heavily on verbal skills, and pictorial aids are utilized. The SSKAT uses a team of evaluators, in an effort to reduce bias and arbitrary decision-making.
2. Thomas-Robert Ames and Perry Samowitz tool (Ames, 1991). This tool assesses the three elements of consent (knowledge, intelligence and voluntariness) using a two-tiered system based on the individual's capacity and mode of expression.
3. Lichtenberg and Strzepek tool (Lichtenberg and Strzepek, 1990). This is an assessment tool used to evaluate the competence of demented inpatients to participate in sexual activity that includes:
    A. Patient's Awareness of the Relationship
       • Is the patient aware of who is initiating contact?
       • Does the patient believe that the other person is a spouse and thus acquiesce out of a delusional belief, or are they cognizant of the other's identity and intent?
       • Can the patient state what level of sexual intimacy they would be comfortable with?
    B. Patient's Ability to Avoid Exploitation
       • Is the behavior consistent with formerly held beliefs/values?
       • Does the patient have the capacity to say no to any uninvited sexual contact?
    C. Patient's Awareness of Potential Risks
       • Does the patient realize that this relationship may be time limited (placement on a unit is temporary)?
       • Can the patient describe how they will react when the relationship ends?

Figure 3.1. Standardized Assessments for Competence to Consent to Sexual Activity.

constitute sexual activity, or are they so thought-disordered that they do not understand they are having sex? Does the patient understand that sexual intercourse can result in pregnancy, sexually transmitted disease, etc?

2. Are the patient's motives for participating in sexual activity rational, or are they severely impacted by the patient's delusions and hallucinations? Is the patient able to integrate their sexual desires with their knowledge about sexual activity and rationally come to a decision whether to participate in sexual activity? For example, is the patient responding to command auditory hallucinations from God telling them to have sex in order to save the world? (It is important for the clinician to not inject his or her own values in this analysis of whether a patient's motives are rational, but to remain as objective as possible.)

3. The patient's understanding of sexual terms – penis, vagina, making love, AIDS, pregnancy, birth control, etc.

4. The patient's general functional abilities – the ability to care for one's self, communicate, etc.

5. The patient's competency in other areas – Is the patient able to give informed consent in other areas, such as deciding medical treatment? One study has shown that when a person has been found previously able to give informed consent in a one area, it is more likely that she will be found capable of consenting to sexual contact (Niederbuhl & Morris, 1993). However, competence in one area does not categorically imply competency in all other areas. Using competence in one area to conclude competence in other areas could have negative ramifications – in fact, some jurisdictions have explicitly held that competency in one area is not a valid criterion in determining an individual's capacity to consent to sexual relations.

A mentally ill person's competence to participate in sexual activity may be impaired by deficits in knowledge about sexual matters. Rozensky and Berman (1984) surveyed 61 mentally ill patients in a partial-hospitalization program with diagnoses of schizophrenia, bipolar disorder and borderline personality disorder. Commonly missed questions on the knowledge portion of the survey included errors on anatomy (e.g., "men and women have an anus"; 22% answered incorrectly) sexual functioning (e.g., "men and women ejaculate"; 43% answered incorrectly) and errors regarding sexual behaviors.

Welch & Clements (1996) describe a hospital policy on sexuality for chronic psychiatric patients that was developed at a British Columbia facility. This policy includes a provision that competent patients may have access to private suites on the hospital grounds for the purpose of sexual activity. The policy states (1) a patient shall be presumed capable of consenting and behaving responsibly unless explicit indicators of possible incompetence exist; (2) if indicators of incompetence are present, a competency test shall be applied; (3) when a patient is found incompetent, the patient's treatment plan must be reviewed and changes made that may help the patient capable in the future; (4) patients found incompetent may apply again in one month, and after three successive denials, may appeal to an independent psychiatrist; and (5) patients granted access may have access suspended or revoked, should indicators of incompetence arise.

The competency test mentioned above in (2) includes a three-part examination. The initial phase consists of a mental status examination, looking for defects in attention, memory, language, thought form, thought content, perception, mood or impulse control that are so severe that the patient is unable to consent to sexual activity or behave responsibly. The qualifier "severe enough" is important because psychiatric inpatients tended not to have a totally clear mental status. The second part of the examination requires the patient to demonstrate a factual understanding of the meaning of certain relevant terms (for example, "safe sex"), while the third part requires the patient to demonstrate practical issues and risks of sexual activity (for example, "how is a condom applied?"). Please see chapter eight of this text for further discussion of these policy issues.

Assessing competence to participate in sexual activity naturally leads to the question of what to do with a patient who is incompetent? First and foremost, the patient's treatment plan should address the specific deficits in the patient's functioning that lead to incompetence, and include a plan to attempt to restore competence in this area. Patients that are incompetent based on psychosis should have their psychosis aggressively treated. Patients who lack information on sexual matters should receive education. Of course, there will be some patients, by nature of their severe illness, who will never achieve competence to participate in sexual activity. In this circumstance, the treatment team must balance two competing principles – the need to protect the patient from incompetently participating in sexual activity, and the patient's right to the least restrictive alternative of care. For example, it would not be permissible to permanently restrict the patient to a locked inpatient ward in order to protect them from incompetently participating in sexual activity. Appropriate safeguards must be devised that both allow the patient to reside in the least restrictive treatment setting, while also taking into account their incompetence.

Another controversial issue has to do with the notification of other competent patients that the incompetent patient will inevitably come into contact with. Other inpatients cannot be expected to know which patients are incompetent to participate in sexual activity, and to chose to approach only competent patients. Yet, confidentiality concerns would not permit informing other patients that this patient is incompetent to participate in sex. The treatment team must develop a plan that will protect the incompetent patient without violating their confidentiality.

Competence to Give Informed Consent to Birth Control

Strong opinions exist regarding incompetent women bearing children. Some have gone so far as to suggest criminal prosecution of women who incompetently consent to sexual activity, and advocate forced birth control methods (*The Seattle Times*, 1991), justifying their position with the opinion that it is wrong to allow children to be born who will be improperly cared for. While this may be an extremist position, women have also been prosecuted for criminally neglecting their children for failing to seek pre-natal care (Gordon, 1987).

Historically, the mentally ill and mentally retarded have been discriminated against regarding their participation in birth control decisions (also see Deegan, chapter 2). The public's view of the mentally retarded as criminally oriented and sexually promiscuous prompted the policies of segregated institutional living arrangements and involuntary sterilizations in the late 1800s and early 1900s. Between 1907 and 1957, roughly 60,000 mentally retarded individuals were sterilized without their consent and/or knowledge (Reed, 1997). Today, experts generally agree that mentally ill and mentally retarded persons have the right to sexual expression, and that sexuality is an inherent need of humans. However, the exact scope of the right of sexual expression remains undefined. Concerns over AIDS, sexual abuse and the lack of sex education for those with mental illness and mental retardation complicate the matter. Respect for the patient's autonomy, a central ethical principle, is especially difficult to implement in the clinical setting of chronic mental illness (McCullough, Coverdale, Bayer & Chervenak, 1992).

There are a variety of possible adverse consequences when a chronically mentally ill patient becomes pregnant (Coverdale, Bayer, McCullough & Chervenak, 1993). Patients who deny pregnancy may receive inadequate prenatal care. Psychotic patients may endanger their health and the outcome of the pregnancy if they act on delusions or auditory hallucinations. Further, children of schizophrenic mothers may be at increased risk for schizophrenia; this risk could approach 45% if the child's father also suffered from schizophrenia. Mentally ill parents may be impaired in their ability to respond to the needs of their children. Women with chronic schizophrenic illnesses, already struggling to maintain contact with reality, may suffer further psychotic regression if faced with the stress involved in either abortion or carrying their pregnancies to term. McEvoy, Hatcher, Appelbaum & Abernethy (1983) reported that chronic schizophrenic womens' factual knowledge and understanding of birth control was extremely limited and that they had many mistaken beliefs about birth control. Psychopathology, manifested in unusual responses and inaccurate answers, frequently disrupted the reasoning of these patients, and could potentially lead to illogical conclusions and imprudent activity. It is logical to conclude that schizophrenic men also bear the same deficits in knowledge and understanding of birth control.

Informed consent for birth control (Grunebaum & Abernethy, 1975) involves three major factors: (1) adequate knowledge on which to base a decision; (2) competence to make a decision; and (3) absence of coercion in the decision-making process. Competence to make such a decision becomes an important issue when the individual is mentally ill and her judgment and reasoning may be impaired. In order to give informed consent, a patient must have the capacity to make a sound judgment and must agree of her own free will to use contraception, knowing its risks and effects.

Analyzing competence to make a decision regarding various birth control methods (oral contraceptives, barrier methods, surgical sterilization and abortion) is similar to the analysis of competence to decide other medical issues, such as taking other medications or undergoing other surgical procedures. That is, the patient must understand the risk and benefits of the proposed medication or procedure, the prognosis with or without undergoing the proposed activity, and the ability to understand alternative methods of treatment. In addition, the patient must be able to understand and use the above information to rationally proceed through the decision-making process.

McCullough *et al.* (1992) suggest that decision-making about healthcare (including birth control issues) can be understood to involve the following process on the part of the patient, a process in which each step presumes successful completion of its predecessors:

1. The patient attends to the information disclosed to him or her by the physician.
2. The patient absorbs, retains and recalls the information disclosed.
3. The patient appreciates that this information has significance in the patient's life and the lives of others. This requires that the patient understands that decisions about health care have consequences for the future and reasons well enough to connect present decisions with future possible consequences. This can be called *cognitive understanding* and requires some nominally intact cognitive abilities.
4. The patient evaluates those consequences on the basis of her values and beliefs. This can be called *evaluative understanding* and requires some nominally integrated sense of oneself.
5. The patient at some meaningful level expresses or communicates both cognitive and evaluative understanding.
6. The patient should be able at some meaningful level to express or communicate a decision based on such understanding.

McCullough *et al.* (1992) further report that for patients with chronic mental illness, one or more of the capacities described above is likely to be impaired and that this is a permanent feature of the mental illness. In addition, this impairment may vary for each of the steps to differing degrees, including differing degrees over time in the same patient. This clinical phenomena is termed *chronically and variably impaired autonomy*. Put another way, a chronically mentally ill patient may at any one time be above the threshold for one capacity (e.g., to attend to what is being said) but below the threshold for another capacity.

Each of the patient's potential areas of deficit in participating in the informed consent process should be assessed, and reversible barriers to the patient's competency should be identified (Coverdale *et al.*, 1993). For example, the patient's comment that she does not believe in birth control may be consistent with values she has previously communicated, or may reflect a simple lack of understanding of contraceptive methods and likely side effects. This lack of understanding could be addressed through education. Her comment may also reflect a paranoia secondary to psychosis. This symptom may in turn impair her ability to attend to, retain and recall information about family planning, as well as to communicate cognitive or evaluative understanding. Patients should receive treatment for symptoms and conditions underlying the variable nature of impaired competency to maximize their ability to provide informed consent. This treatment should be tailored to meet the specific needs of the patient and to address the specific areas of incompetence.

There are various legal models as to how to best proceed if a patient lacks competence to participate in birth control issues. The first model involves the concept of "substituted judgment," which is what the incompetent person would want, if they were competent. This differs from the "best interests" model, which takes into account what is best for the patient, regardless of what the patient would have wanted if they were competent. The third model involves seeking the input of a substitute decision-maker, such as the patient's family. One appellate court in New York (*In the Matter of Barbara C.*, 1984) ruled that a mentally ill incompetent woman's family should decide if she should have an abortion. The hospital sought not to have the woman's family decide, but asked the court to determine what the incompetent woman herself would have done if she were competent (substituted judgment). However, a Massachusetts appellate court did follow the substituted judgment model – determining what the incompetent would have wanted if competent (*In the Matter of Jane A.*, 1994). Other states, such as Louisiana, have utilized a best interest model (*Causeway Medical Suite v. Ieyoub*, 1997).

It is important to appreciate that competence, over the course of time, may fluctuate. As a patient's level of impairment from their illness waxes and wanes over time, so does their competency. As a general rule, fluctuating competency equates with incompetence, and the local statutes regarding how to proceed in the face of incompetence should be invoked. Substitute decision-makers may wish to utilize long-acting but reversible methods of birth control (such as Norplant)

for patients whose competence fluctuates over time. This insures that
the patient's wishes may be adhered to if her competence returns in
the future.

Competence to Parent and to Relinquish Parental Rights

Persons with mental illness have normal desires to procreate and parent children. Pregnancies that result in live births among seriously
mentally ill persons may raise the question of who is to care for the
child? When the parents are seriously mentally ill, this question may
put in direct conflict two competing principles – the parents right to
raise the child in a manner they choose, versus the child's right to be
raised in a caring environment that promotes the child's best interests. All states have statutes governing the removal of a child from a
parent's custody due to neglect or abuse. In Ohio, for example, a neglected child (Ohio Revised Code 2151.03) includes any child: (1) who
is abandoned by his parents; (2) who lacks adequate parental care
because of the faults or habits of the child's parents; (3) whose parents neglect the child or refuse to provide proper or necessary subsis-
tence, education, medical or surgical care, or other care necessary for
the child's health, morals or well being; (4) whose parents neglect the
child or refuse to provide the special care made necessary by the child's
mental condition; (5) who, because of the omission of the parents,
suffers physical or mental injury that harms or threatens to harm the
child's health or welfare; or (6) who is subjected to out-of-home care
child neglect. While certainly a large number of mentally ill persons
are fit parents, it is feasible to envision each of the above circumstances
as a reality with a seriously mentally ill parent, caused by the parent's
delusion, disorganized thoughts or prominent negative symptoms.

If a court makes the legal determination that a child is indeed neglected, the next step is for the court to determine the proper disposi-
tion of the child (Grisso, 1986). The court must determine if the child
can be adequately protected by allowing the child to continue to live
with the parent(s) under the supervision of social service agents, or
whether placement in a foster home is required. All states have statutes that allow the court to permanently severe the ties between a
parent and a child under certain circumstances – these statutes usually require a finding that a parent is incompetent or unfit to provide
satisfactorily for the child's welfare. The threshold of evidence regarding the need for termination of parental rights may vary with a
jurisdiction's philosophy concerning the rights of natural parents.
Smith (1979) classified these statues as: (1) parental rights jurisdictions (often requiring strong proof of unfitness in order to justify termination); (2) child-focused jurisdictions (which attended primarily
to the importance of alternatives for the welfare of the child); and (3)
jurisdictions with positions intermediate between the first two. If the

court determines that the parent is unfit, the child may be adopted permanently over parental objections.

THE RELATIONSHIP BETWEEN LEGAL INSANITY
AND SERIOUS MENTAL ILLNESS

Traditionally, a crime consists of two elements: a forbidden act (actus reus) and a guilty mind (mens rea). For example, if a defendant intentionally strikes another, he is guilty of a battery. In this example the actus reus is the striking of the victim, while the mens rea is the defendant's intention to strike the victim. (There are exceptions to this rule. Some crimes require only that an actus reus occur without mens rea. These crimes are called strict liability crimes. For example, statutory rape requires only that the defendant commit the act of participating in sexual activity with a minor, regardless of whether the defendant knew that his sexual partner was a minor.) The requirement that a crime consists of both actus reus and mens rea is based on the social policy that punishment for an act should depend primarily on the *intent* of the wrongdoer, with less weight give to the *result* of his/her actions.

The concept of Not Guilty by Reason of Insanity has its origins in the principle of mens rea, and dates as far back as ancient Greece (Robinson, 1996). Simply put, a wrongdoer with a mental illness that causes him to commit an offense while believing he is doing the right thing (or without the ability to resist taking action) lack mens rea, and is not held responsible. In the Middle Ages, under early English common law a wrongdoer was not held responsible for his actions if he was globally unable to distinguish right from wrong. Later, this concept became more refined, and defendants were excused from their illegal acts if their mental disease made them unable to ascertain that the specific act in question was wrong, or they were unable to refrain from committing the act.

Most jurisdictions in the United States currently utilize insanity standards that are a variant on two themes: the McNaughten standard and the Model Penal Code. The McNaughten standard arose from an English murder trial in 1843 in which Daniel McNaughten was accused of murdering Edward Drummond, the secretary to Prime Minister Sir Robert Peel. McNaughten's intended target was Prime Minister Peel, but he mistook Drummond for Peel. McNaughten was laboring under a paranoid delusional system that included the belief that he was persecuted by the political party that Peel led. McNaughten was eventually determined by the court to be insane, and the resultant public outrage led the appellate court to formulate a new standard for insanity, now called the McNaughten standard. This standard requires that, at the time of the offense, a defendant have a mental disease or defect so severe as to cause him not to know the wrongfulness of his illegal act, or not to know the nature and quality of the act.

Beginning in 1955, the Model Penal Code (a series of model statutes that some states have adopted portions of) articulated a standard for insanity. This standard states that a defendant is not responsible for his conduct if, at the time of the offense, as a result of mental disease or defect, he lacks substantial capacity to either: (1) appreciate the wrongfulness of his conduct, or; (2) conform his conduct to the requirements of the law.

The question that naturally arises when utilizing either the McNaughten standard or Model Penal Code standard is which psychiatric diagnoses qualify as a "mental disease or defect" for the purposes of legal insanity? Most statutes do not specify which diagnoses are included, and it has been left to courts to interpret this standard. Certainly, most psychotic and mood disorders would quality, such as schizophrenia or bipolar disorder. Courts have usually not interpreted the standard to allow personality disorders, substance use disorders, or paraphilias to satisfy as a mental disease or defect for the purposes of insanity, even though they are valid DSM-IV diagnoses. The following example illustrates this point:

Mr. J. was a 50 year old man with a long history of schizophrenia. He had the chronic delusion that women he encountered while walking in public gave him sexually stimulating signals. For example, he believed that when a woman licked her lips or looked at him, she wanted to have sex with him. Mr. J. never acted on these signals, but always simply kept walking down the sidewalk. He believed that these women transmitted sexually stimulating signals to him via telepathy. After receiving these signals he usually found a public restroom and masturbated. He never approached the objects of his delusions or spoke with them. He had a history of multiple psychiatric hospitalizations and noncompliance with antipsychotic medication.

Mr. J. also had a history of sexual fantasies involving children, usually girls from the age of three to ten years old. He frequently fantasized about young children while masturbating, and children that lived in close proximity to him on occasion told their parents that Mr. J. had spoken lewdly to them or masturbated in their presence.

Mr. J. was charged with one count of Gross Sexual Imposition, stemming from the accusation that he kissed a six-year-old girl and fondled her buttocks while in a bowling alley. When referred for an insanity evaluation, he told the examiner that he had been compliant with his medications around the time of the offense, and he experienced no unusual psychiatric symptoms during the offense. He reported that he gave the victim five dollars because it made him feel good to help others, and that he kissed and fondled the girl because "she wanted it." Mr. J. said he had not received any sexual signals from the victim, and she had not transmitted any telepathic signals to him. After kissing and fondling the victim, Mr. J. immediately left the bowling alley because "her mother might find out." The victim indeed told her mother, who called police.

Mr. J. initially denied any involvement with the victim when questioned by police, but soon made a confession.

This example illustrates the distinction between conduct caused by the defendant's schizophrenia as opposed to conduct caused by his pedophilia. While the law may not hold him responsible for actions which were motivated by his schizophrenic delusions, clearly the defendant's behavior in the above incident was motivated by his pedophilia, not his schizophrenia. Because the law does not interpret "mental disease or defect" to include pedophilia, Mr. J. was not eligible for a finding of Not Guilty by Reason of Insanity.

Separate from the question of which diagnoses qualify as a mental disease or defect for the purposes of insanity, both the McNaughten rule and the Model Penal Code have additional requirements for a finding of legal insanity. In the case of the McNaughten standard, the defendant's mental disease or defect must have caused him not to know the wrongfulness of his actions at the time of the offense. In other words, the defendant's mental disorder must cause him to believe his actions are legally or morally correct (legal versus moral correctness varies according to the jurisdiction). The most frequently encountered offenses that result in legal insanity (using the McNaughten rule) are those perpetrated by a psychotic offender with persecutory delusions that result in the defendant acting in perceived self defense (Pinals & Noffsinger, 1997). For example, a defendant who delusionally believes that his neighbor is about to kill him and shoots the neighbor in self defense would be likely to receive an insanity verdict. This stems from the fact that if the circumstances of his delusions were actually occurring (that his neighbor actually is about to kill him), the defendant would be justified in his actions. In the case of the Model Penal Code rule, the defendant's mental disorder must cause him to lack substantial capacity to either: (1) appreciate the wrongfulness of his conduct (also known as the cognitive arm, similar to the McNaughten rule), or; (2) conform his conduct to the requirements of the law (also known as the volitional arm).

Offenses of a sexual nature (rape, gross sexual imposition) are far more likely to result in an insanity finding under the Model Penal Code rule's volitional arm, as compared to the cognitive arm of the Model Penal Code or the McNaughten rule. This is because it is unlikely that a defendant will be laboring under a delusion that would cause him to believe that forcing another to have sexual contact with him would be the right thing to do. In comparison, a defendant would be more likely to have a delusional system that would cause him to be unable to refrain from committing the offense. The following example illustrates this point:

Mr. R. was a 42-year-old man with a 20-year history of schizophrenia. He was charged with the rape of his neighbor, an elderly woman. Mr. R. stopped taking his antipsychotic medication three months prior to the offense, due to extrapyramidal side effects. Beginning one month prior to the offense he experienced command auditory hallucinations of God's voice telling him that he was a prophet, and that he must have sexual intercourse in order to impregnate a woman who would bear the new Christ. The voices also told Mr. R. that if he failed to impregnate a woman by midnight on the day of the offense, the world would come to an end. On the day of the offense Mr. R. was very distressed, because he had been unable to find a willing sexual partner, despite many attempts over the past several weeks. He called the police and told them the world was going to end, but the police dispatcher instructed him to stop making prank telephone calls. Believing there was only fifteen minutes before the world was going to end, he broke into the victim's apartment and forcibly had sexual intercourse with her. Upon the arrival of the police, Mr. R. was lying on the victim's floor, and mumbled "We are safe – the new savior has been conceived."

This example illustrates a delusional system that most likely would qualify for legal insanity under the volitional arm of the Model Penal Code. After exhausting other methods to achieve his goal of conceiving the new Christ and preventing the end of the world (finding willing sexual partners and calling the police), and under time pressure to stop the world from ending, Mr. R. believed he was left with only one option, which was to break into his neighbor's apartment and commit the offense.

EVALUATING SEXUAL ASSAULTS IN THE HOSPITAL

Sexual assaults involving hospitalized seriously mentally ill patients are relatively common occurrences, and frequently result in strong emotional reactions among hospital staff, patients and the general public. Sexual assaults can occur between two patients, a patient perpetrator and staff victim, or less frequently, a staff perpetrator and patient victim. Sexual assaults can occur as the result of severe delusions or in response to command auditory hallucinations. Sexual assaults can also occur in patients with severe disturbances in thought process, such as very disorganized patients. Patients with manic features, impulse control difficulties or dementia also can commit sexual assaults.

Given the requirement that hospitals must afford patients the least restrictive conditions of treatment, chronically institutionalized patients are often afforded increasingly permissive privileges, such as grounds privileges or off-grounds passes. As the level of freedom increases, staff supervision and observation decreases. Assaults on other patients can occur when the patient is free of staff supervision while on grounds privileges, or can less frequently occur on the inpatient unit itself.

When an assault occurs, the police or hospital security should be called, and statements should be taken from the alleged perpetrator, victim, and witnesses. The hospital administration and security personnel should work with the local prosecutor and victim to determine if criminal charges will be filed. Some prosecutors are hesitant to file criminal charges against a seriously mentally ill patient, because of the relatively small chance that the defendant will be convicted, and the more likely outcome that the defendant will be found Incompetent to Stand Trial or legally insane. The prosecutor should undertake an analysis of the severity of the charges balanced with the likely outcome of trial, in order to determine whether prosecution is desirable. However, prosecutors often erroneously conclude that a finding of Incompetence to Stand Trial or Not Guilty by Reason of Insanity is an undesirable outcome, which is not necessarily accurate. A defendant who is ultimately found insane will be placed under the jurisdiction of the criminal court, and will have to comply with conditions set by the court, such as mandatory medication compliance or supervised living arrangements after eventual discharge from the hospital. Often, defendants found Incompetent to Stand Trial for major assaults face the same court-imposed conditions. In addition, the hospital administration should not elect to abandon prosecution of the perpetrator based on the unlikely chances of conviction, for the hospital administration would be overstepping their role and invading an area reserved for courts and juries.

Regardless of the decision of whether to prosecute or not, the hospital's clinical staff should evaluate the alleged perpetrator to determine whether a more restrictive treatment setting is required, such as a maximum security hospital. A through assessment for violence risk factors should be completed, and any identified risk factors should be addressed in the patient's treatment plan.

Hospital staff committing sexual assaults or engaging in sexual activity with patients is an especially contentious topic. The most frequent scenario is a hospital employee with sociopathic traits engaging in sexual behavior with a patient who is incompetent to consent to sexual activity. This incompetence stems from the patient's mental illness and/or mental retardation, as well as the inherent coercive nature of the staff/patient relationship. Mental health clinicians, be it physicians, psychologists, nurses or mental health technicians, should never engage in a sexual relationship with current or former patients. The imbalance of power in a therapist/patient relationship and strong transferences involved make sexual activity with a patient inappropriate. When patient/staff sexual activity does occur, an extra layer of assessment of the situation should be undertaken, as the hospital administration could potentially face a conflict of interest in their dual roles as employer of the alleged perpetrator and caretaker of the patient. An independent evaluation from an external clinical is often helpful, to determine whether the patient's treatment needs in light of the staff/patient sexual activity are adequately being addressed.

It is clear that the issues of sexuality in persons with mental illness are complex. At present, there is only limited legal guidance on these matters.

REFERENCES

Ames, T.H. (1991). Guidelines for providing sexuality-related services to severely and profoundly retarded individuals: the challenge for the nineteen-nineties. *Sexuality and Disability* 9:113–122.

Causeway Medical Suite et al., v. Ieyoub et al., 109 F.3d 1096 (1997).

Coverdale, J.H., Bayer, T.L., McCullough, L.B. & Chervenak, F.A. (1993). Respecting the autonomy of chronic mentally ill women in decisions about contraception. *Hospital and Community Psychiatry* 44:671–674.

Dusky v. United States 362:U.S. 402, 80 S. Ct. 788 (1960).

Forced birth control? Drug abusers not mentally competent to make decisions (editorial) (1991, July 2). *The Seattle Times* p. A7.

Gordon, L. (1987). Reproductive rights for today; some policy proposals. *The Nation* 245:230.

Grisso, T. (1986). *Evaluating competencies.* New York: Plenum Press.

Grunebaum, H. & Abernethy, V. (1975). Ethical issues in family planning for hospitalized psychiatric patients. *American Journal of Psychiatry* 132:236–240.

Gutheil, T.G. (1997). *Competence: Civil and Criminal.* Presentation at the 28th Annual Meeting of American Academy of Psychiatry and the Law, Denver, CO.

In the Matter of Barbara C., 101 A.D. 2d 137, 474 N.Y.S. 2d 799 (1984).

In the Matter of Jane A. 36 Mass. App. Ct. 236, 629 N.E. 2d 1337 (1994).

Jones, G.H. (1995). Informed consent in chronic schizophrenia? *British Journal of Psychiatry* 167:565–568.

Lichtenberg, P.A. & Strzepek, D.M. (1990). Assessments of institutionalized dementia patients' competencies to participate in intimate relationships. *The Gerontologist* 30:117–120.

McCullough, L.B., Coverdale, J.H., Bayer, T.L. & Chervenak, F.A. (1992). Ethically justified guidelines for family planning interventions to prevent pregnancy for female patients with chronic mental illness. *American Journal of Obstetrics and Gynecology* 167:19–25.

McEvoy, J.P., Hatcher, A., Appelbaum, P.S. & Abernethy, V. (1983). Chronic schizophrenic women's attitudes toward sex, pregnancy, birth control, and childrearing. *Hospital and Community Psychiatry* 34:536–539.

Niederbuhl, J.M. & Morris, C.D. (1993). Sexual knowledge and the capability of persons with dual diagnosis to consent to sexual contact. *Sexuality and Disability* 11:295–307.

Ohio Revised Code section 2151.03.

Pinals, D. & Noffsinger, S.G. (1997). *Characterization of symptoms in NGRI patients.* Presentation at the 28th Annual Meeting of American Academy of Psychiatry and the Law, Denver, CO.

Rape conviction overturned. (1983, October 20). *The Associated Press* (news release).

Reed, E.J. (1997). Criminal law and the capacity of mentally retarded persons to consent to sexual activity. *Virginia Law Review* 83:799–827.

Robinson, D.N. (1996). *Wild beasts and idle humours: The insanity defense from antiquity to the present.* Cambridge: Harvard University Press.

Rozensky, R.H. & Berman, C. (1984). Sexual knowledge, attitudes, and experiences of chronic psychiatric patients. *Psychosocial Rehabilitation Journal* 721–27.

Smith, S. (1979). Psychological parents vs. biological parents: The courts' responses to new directions in child custody dispute resolutions. *Journal of Family Law* 17:545–585.

Welch, S.J. & Clements, G.W. (1996). Development of a policy on sexuality for hospitalized chronic psychiatric patients. *Canadian Journal of Psychiatry* 41:273–279.

Wyatt v. Stickney, 344 F. Supp. 373 (1972).

4

Dilemmas of Managing Sexual Activity Among Psychiatric Patients

PETER F. BUCKLEY, MICHAEL HOGAN,
DALE P. SVENDSEN and GEORGE GINTOLI

INPATIENT SEXUALITY AND THE BALANCE OF RESPONSIBILITIES

State mental hospitals have undergone dramatic changes in the past 10 years (Bachrach, 1996; Hogan, 1996). The closing of institutions, the coalescing of services and the (by and large) greater continuity of care between inpatient and community providers have dominated public psychiatry and have resulted in improved standards of care within most state facilities. Allied to these developments have been the prodigious advances in the pharmacological treatment of psychosis, which have vastly improved the quality of life and expectations for sustained community tenure among those patients who hithertofore would have resided indefinitely in long-term facilities (Buckley, 1998). The public mental health system has also been responsive to broader developments in health care that presage the arrival of managed care approaches, an open-market, competitive philosophy and consumer choice. These competitive forces require that state facilities *at a minimum* provide active treatment (as opposed to the historical and often too true stereotype of custodial care) and that they focus on objective patient outcomes (Imbornoni *et al.*, 1997). Changes in the patterns of care are results of interrelated trends: improved treatments, expanded community care, and expanded financial support for inpatient care in other settings such as general hospitals. These changes are also linked to changing attitudes about

53

mental illness (e.g., support for mental health's inclusion in health reform as reported by the Judge David I. Bazelon Center for Mental Health Law, 1995) and changing paradigms of illness such as the "recovery paradigm" (Anthony, 1993). These changes have reduced the capacity of state hospitals. But these facilities still serve a crucial role and treat many vulnerable patients. Bachrach has suggested that amidst such change, state facilities have the opportunity to redefine and assert their role as a resource and also their expertise in the management (both clinical and policy making) of patients with serious mental illness (Bachrach, 1996). Viewed in this context, endeavors to promote thoughtful and sensible deliberation on inpatient sexuality are both timely and necessary.

However, this is certainly not an easy charge (see Figure 4.1). Inpatient sexuality is, in contrast to the voluminous literature on aggression and suicidal behaviors, a remarkably neglected topic. One can assume that this is, in large part, due to the contentious and affect-laden nature of this issue. Also, it reflects the impossible dilemmas imposed upon hospitals. Balancing the sexual rights of inpatients with the complex institutional responsibilities is, at best, difficult and, at worst, untenable (Buckley & Hyde, 1997). Psychiatric facilities are simultaneously required to uphold patients' rights and privacy, to protect vulnerable patients, and to be responsive to the prevailing social norms. Historically, hospitals have been blamed for failing on all three counts. In an era that medicalized the sexuality of psychiatric patients (Achtar & Thompson, 1980), the occurrence of sexual activity in psychiatric

Mental Health Related Factors
- delusions, hallucinations, thought disorder
- negative symptoms (apathy, amotivation, anhedonia)
- social skills deficits
- cognitive deficits
- medication-induced sexual dysfunction
- insight and competency
- self-esteem, value

Sociopolitical Factors
- mental illness stigma and myths about reproduction
- human rights, sexual freedom, desire
- Americans with Disabilities (ADA) law
- legal protection of vulnerable persons
- institutional liability

Figure 4.1. Contextual Factors of Sexuality Among Persons with Mental Illness.

facilities was viewed as evidence of the uncontrollable psychic urges; these were often considered as causative factors in major mental illness (Vandereycken, 1993). This perspective legitimized the devaluing of intimacy and sexuality among persons with serious mental illness (Chase, 1988). Alleged sexual incidents between patients were the subject of public outcry. These were highlighted as incontrovertible evidence of the undesirable state of care in long-stay psychiatric facilities. Threatened by hostile public opinion and lacking direction in the absence of policies, hospital staff were (explicitly and implicitly) encouraged to minimize the sexual practices of inpatients.

Holbrook provides a chilling account of these dynamics (Holbrook, 1989). At a New York facility, the failure to report a sexual incident (at the request of the apparently consenting patient) unleashed intense and persistent scrutiny by legal and public agencies. Staff were subsequently instructed, under fear of censure, to report all incidents of sexual activity. All such incidents were then investigated with the vigor of a medieval inquisition. Not surprisingly, this led to increased notification of sexual activity among inpatients. This further fueled public scorn. There were claims that the institution was being mismanaged. Staff morale declined. Staff pursued repeated investigations under duress, with the threat that any error of judgement could result in dismissal. Patient's privacy was infringed upon. Patients were subject to repeated questioning by various hospital staff and, potentially, by external police, detectives and even the district attorney. Holbrook highlights, parenthetically, that of the hundreds of investigations of sexual or physical assault following the initial incident only one or two patients were actually prosecuted. Additionally, the commission established to provide recommendations on this issue became concerned that major crimes and patient injustices would now go undetected because of voluminous reports of minor crimes. Despite the concerted efforts of everybody involved, it seemed as if the pendulum had swung – and was firmly wedged – in the opposite direction (Holbrook, 1989).

Subsequent events have thrown this health and administrative dilemma of patient sexuality into sharper relief. The risk of spreading HIV infection among psychiatric patients necessitated examination of the sexual practices of this group (Grassi, 1996). There was also a pressing need to identify and protect vulnerable patients. At the same time, the growth of advocacy and recovery movements have promoted the concept of normalization and freedom of expression among persons with serious mental illness (see Deegan, this volume). Additionally, public expression and acceptance of sexuality has changed dramatically over the past 15 years. The same can be said, albeit to a lesser extent, for the public awareness and understanding of serious mental illness itself. While the challenges for psychiatric facilities in dealing with patient sexuality remain the same (promote normalization, protect patients, uphold official and social mores), it may be argued that the context in which these duties prevail is substantially different now.

Sex and Institutional Subculture

Despite counterclaims and vigorous denials, it is clear that some patients within long-term psychiatric facilities engage in sexual activity. As is the case in any other community, behavior is in part shaped and/or regulated by the prevailing subculture. There has been effectively no research to determine which elements modulate an institutional subculture to be either permissive, promoting, or antagonistic towards sexual expression among inpatients. It is overly simplistic to equate sexual activity among inpatients with inadequate administrative management of the hospital (Holbrook, 1989). It is more likely that several factors, relating to both patients and staff, interact in a complex fashion. For instance, it is apparent (both from the literature and clinical experience) that the type of diagnosis and the level of illness acuity among patients on any unit influence the extent and pattern of sexual expression. In general, there is less overt sexual behavior between patients on an acute unit. This is in large part due to the severity of illness. Most patients are too unwell and actively psychotic to engage in intimate (sexual) relationships at that time. On the other hand, long-stay units vary in sexual activity as a function of the diagnostic categories. In their analysis of staff perceptions of inpatient sexuality, Civic and colleagues (1993) noted differences in sexual expression across hospital units. Staff from all-male units stated that intercourse between males was common [no figures were provided]. Staff from the geriatric units reported that patients rarely had intercourse but that they engaged in masturbation. It was recorded that sex in exchange for material items such as cigarettes or food occurred on all units. Sexual bartering has also been recorded between patients in the community (Cournos *et al.*, 1994; Coverdale *et al.*, 1993). This behavior is, therefore, not solely a function of the availability of goods within hospitals. This behavior may in turn be related to predatory and victimization patterns among patients in hospital. Higher functioning patients are apt to exploit lower functioning patients directly by forced sexual advances and by intimidation. Such behavior is particularly distressing for hospital staff who are often genuinely unsure as to how to manage this problem (Civic *et al.*, 1993). It has been emphasized earlier in this chapter (and elsewhere throughout this book) that staff attitudes towards sexuality are an important aspect of this dilemma (Mossman *et al.*, 1997; Cohen and Tanenbaum, 1985). The response of staff may range from ignorance to (covert) permissiveness to authoritarian refusal of any expression of human intimacy. The predominant attitude in the unit will prevail in the absence of firm administrative direction on inpatient sexuality.

Sexual expression may also vary according to whether the unit is single sex or co-ed in composition. This is an important consideration on acute units. The presence of female patients may increase arousal in young male acutely psychotic patients who have sexual delusions (and vice versa). There is also heightened risk of sexual activity for those patients who are impulsive and sexually disinhibited. The impact of co-ed versus single sex units in long-stay hospitals is less clear. Sexual relationships are not exclusive to patients on their own ward and are more likely to be widely distributed throughout the hospital. In a study of sexual activity among patients in state facilities (Buckley & Hyde, 1997; also, see below) 50 out of 57 hospitals reported that sexual behavior was a problem. Thirty-four hospitals were exclusively co-ed and 8 had exclusively single sex units. Fifteen had a mixture of single sex and co-ed units. The extent of inpatient sexuality in this study did not differ as a function of unit composition.

Balancing Administrative Responsibilities: The Example of Smoking

Smoking by psychiatric inpatients provides an excellent example of the complexities of addressing normal human behavior within the institutional setting. Rates of smoking among patients with schizophrenia are much higher than rates in the general population or in other psychiatric groups. DeLeon and colleagues (1995) reported that 85% of all patients with a diagnosis of schizophrenia in a state hospital were smokers compared with a rate of 67% among all other diagnostic groups. High rates of smoking among long-stay patients have been attributed to chronic boredom due to institutionalization. However, recent evidence suggests that there may also be a strong biological relationship between smoking and schizophrenia (Dalack *et al.*, 1996). Hospital administrations often pursue a no-smoking policy to promote healthy lifestyles, to limit physical morbidity among inpatients, to minimize fire risks, to curtail any predatory or exploitative behaviors that may be associated with smoking; and, inevitably, to achieve compliance with standards set by federal and other accreditation bodies.

It has been shown that prohibition of smoking on acute units can be achieved without any significant or sustained impact on either patient's symptoms or on unit functioning. However, the regulation of cigarette smoking in long-stay facilities is more problematic. In particular, it raises serious human rights dilemmas not dissimilar to those of sexuality in inpatients. An absolute ban on smoking may drastically reduce the rate of smoking (assuming that there is a strong administrative ruling and also staff acceptance). However, this may also promote a covert smoking subculture within the hospital. This subculture is characterized by disregard for the smoking policy and by exploitation of vulnerable patients. Bartering for cigarettes becomes commonplace. Cigarettes may be used as currency for food, clothing, or sexual intimacy. Smoking may occur in concealed locations that are fire hazards. Additionally, human rights advocates deplore the prohibition of smoking as a serious infringement of personal liberty. Hospital staff (particularly those who smoke are often sympathetic to this issue of patient rights) may be unwilling to enforce a stringent policy. On the other hand, if smoking by patients goes unchecked, the health safety and safety risks are untenable. Administrative neglect of this issue places both patients and staff at risk. As with issue of inpatient sexuality, hospital policies on smoking are required to be both sensible and sensitive. Implementation of policies must be consistent across units and between each clinical discipline. The same can be said for the management of inpatient sexuality.

Hospital Policies on Sexual Activity

In the absence of administrative direction, staff can feel bewildered and forced to resort to their personal beliefs and intuition in handling difficult circumstances and sexual incidents. Moreover, idiosyncratic or personalized responses may contradict the responses of other team members and result in role confusion, inconsistency, and fragmentation of the team process (Kreitner & Grof, 1981). Administrative directives should provide both the philosophical guidance to staff and, perhaps more importantly, explicit and pragmatic instructions that assist staff to be able to deal immediately and thereafter with sexual incidents as they occur either on the unit or elsewhere on the hospital grounds. Irrespective of the ultimate outcome, inconsistency across patient assessments and/or failure to adopt a standardized and balanced approach to the management of sexual incidents exposes a hospital to the risk of liability. It is clear that, in any given institution, there is a diversity of opinion among staff as to whether patients should or should not engage in sexual activity (Cohen & Tanenbaum, 1985; Welch et al., 1991; also see Welch et al., this volume). There is even more dissent among staff as to how such circumstances should be managed (Civic et al.,1993). In a survey of 70 inpatient psychiatric units in Canada (Kreitner & Grof, 1981), 20% of respondents reported that relationships were supported by staff. Forty-five percent described using management approaches that included confrontation, individual therapy, group discussion, staff discussion, common sense, and discharge of the patients involved (a strategy that is also likely to be used in other facilities). In a subsequent report of staff attitudes to sexual activity among inpatients (Civic et al., 1993), staff listed the lack of a hospital policy as a major impediment to the effective clinical management of sexual behavior. This was also viewed as a significant contributory factor to the occupational distress experienced by staff with this issue. This confusion is also very stressful for persons in treatment (see Deegan, this book). Kreitner and Grof (1981) were astonished to find that not a single psychiatric unit among 70 facilities had a written policy on sexuality among inpatients. Welch and Clements reported that the situation was largely unchanged some 15 years later (Welch & Clements, 1996). They put together a multidisciplinary team to develop a policy that would facilitate and administrate the practice of consensual sex among inpatients at their hospital (Welch & Clements, 1996). The formation of this policy and the outcome for the hospital are described in the chapter in this book by these authors.

With regard to the U.S., little is known about the extent and the content of policies in state facilities that might govern the sexual practices of inpatients. To obtain a clear understanding of the issues and responses to the sexual behavior of inpatients, we devised and circulated a survey to the directors of 86 state psychiatric facilities located in Ohio, North Carolina, South Carolina, New Jersey, New York, Pennsylvania, South Dakota, Tennessee, Texas, and Washington (Buckley & Hyde, 1997). The hospitals surveyed were predominately acute and long-stay facilities whose patient populations were broadly similar to the population of our hospital, in which patients with severe psychosis were overrepresented. The questionnaire comprised four questions: whether the hospital had a formal policy on sexual behavior of patients, the extent to which such behavior was viewed as problematic or clinically relevant, whether a psychoeducational program existed to deal with this behavior, and whether the hospital had mixed- or single-sex units. Respondents were encouraged to include any comments at the end of the questionnaire.

Fifty-seven questionnaires were returned. This yielded a respectable response rate of 66 percent. Forty-seven of the 57 respondents (83%) reported that they had some policy relating to sexual behavior among patients. Eighty-eight percent stated that sexual activity between inpatients was a problem at their facility. Seventy-five percent of the facilities that were surveyed reported having psychoeducational activities to address sexual behavior. Some respondents gave examples of the context of their sexual programs (e.g., HIV prevention, prenatal care, intimacy relationships). Some policies addressed only specific areas of patient sexuality (i.e., sexual assault, HIV prevention). Although a definite concern was expressed in the respondents' comments, it seemed as if many facilities were just beginning to consider this issue. The findings of this study are summarized in Table 4.1.

These results provide indirect evidence (in the context of a heretofore surprising dearth of formal information) that some patients in state psychiatric facilities are sexually active. Additionally, it appeared from this study that many facilities have developed at least some form of policy to address this issue. In total, 50 of 57 respondents indicated that sexual activity between patients occurred at their facility. However,

Table 4.1. Sexual Activity and Responses in State Hospitals.*

Issue	Hospital Response
Existence of hospital policy (yes/no)	47/10
Sexual Behavior	
Considered an ongoing problem	15
Considered an infrequent problem	35
Not considered a problem	7
Existence of a psychoeducation program (yes/no)	43/14
Psychiatric Units	
Co-ed units	34
Single sex units	8
Both co-ed units and single sex units	15

* See Buckley and Hyde (1997)

the survey was brief (so as to encourage response) and no details were solicited on the extent, frequency, or pattern of sexual behavior among inpatients. It is plausible that the rate of sexual activity was underestimated since the questionnaire was completed (presumably) without recourse to any formal evaluation of sexuality at each facility. Additionally, 29 of the original 86 directors of hospitals who were sampled did not return the questionnaire. It is possible that some of these facilities had significant difficulties with this issue and therefore chose not to complete the survey. The introductory letter specified that the survey was anonymous and that information would be treated as confidential. Nevertheless, cognizant of the risks of disclosure of sexual incidents in the hospital setting (Holbrook, 1989), some facilities may have been reluctant to participate. It should be noted, however, that the 66% response rate is actually very acceptable for this form of research (Johnson *et al.*, 1992). We speculate that disinterest, apathy, or communication problems (e.g., loss of the questionnaire) were the most likely explanations for the incomplete study sample. The brevity of the survey is likely to have enhanced the response rate. However, this is at the sacrifice of the quality of information obtained. For example, although 83% of respondents reported having a policy that addressed inpatient sexuality we did not obtain details on these policies.

There is little available information on actual hospital policies on sexuality. The policy developed by Kreitner and Grof (1981) following their review of a Canadian hospital consisted of a simple, philosophical statement: "The ward has both male and female patients. Some patients develop emotional and/or sexual attachment to each other, partly due to the amount of time spent together in the same place. As this ward is a closed environment, we ask that you respect the feelings and moral standards of other patients by not engaging in sexual activity of any kind on the units. If you develop a relationship with another patient, staff will get together with you to help decide whether this relationship is beneficial or detrimental to you and whether it would be to your advantage to continue or discontinue the relationship." This policy is explicit in its prohibition of sexual activity but does not discriminate between masturbation in privacy and sexual activity between patients. It does, however, acknowledge the broader human context in which these relationships occur. It also pays credence to the potential that relationships may be therapeutic and beneficial.

We have recently conducted a content analysis of policies on sexuality from state facilities. A manuscript describing these policies in detail is under review (Buckley & Robben, submitted for publication) and, accordingly, a brief outline of the findings are reported herein. Thirty-one policies were collected and reviewed. Ten percent were one page or less in length and 23% were documents composed of several related policies. However, surprisingly, less than 60% had either a description of different sexual behaviors discrimination. Many policies were simplistic and failed to even address such fundamental issues as personal autonomy or staff education. These results confirm the impression from our previous study (Buckley & Hyde, 1997) that, while many facilities possess a specific policy on sexuality, more often than not this policy is rudimentary in form and lacks the necessary detail to be of benefit to unit staff.

As advocated earlier (see Introduction), state hospitals now have the opportunity to assert their role in the management of serious and persistent mental illness. The dilemmas of inpatient sexuality are more apt to arise in long-term care facilities where intimate human relationships evolve over the duration of hospital stay. Policies on inpatient sexuality should acknowledge this. Mossman and colleagues (1997) in an excellent review of this issue, offer some important insights on this distinction. Their comments are based on the assumption that hospitals are analogous to public places and, accordingly, should reflect the social norms of expressive behavior and privacy. They conclude that is "reasonable" to request patients on acute care units to refrain from sexual activity and they advocate for policies that clearly state this prohibition for the acute inpatient setting. On the other hand, they highlight the risk of infringement on personal rights and, specifically, the Americans with Disabilities (ADA) law if stringent policies are enforced in long stay facilities. In long stay facilities, they argue cogently, the concept of a public place and social norms' is less applicable. They state: "Long term facilities must respond to different needs and conditions to allow patients dwelling there some opportunity for dignified living."

Policies should encompass the developments in the recovery model and they should stress the importance of fostering personal autonomy. The chapter by Deegan (This book) amplifies and provides guidance on this important point. Additionally, they should be of sufficient detail to provide direction to staff on how to manage sexuality among patients on their unit. This is not only desirable clinically but it is also necessary to obviate unwarranted distress for staff. Staff should not be required to address such complex human behavior without administrative direction. We offer some broad headings that may help to provide a framework for further discussion towards a comprehensive policy (see Figure 4.2). Mossman and colleagues (1997) provide a model policy that covers the following: (1) admission and screening; (2) ability to consent; (3) sex education and contraceptive counselling; (4) masturbation; (5) consensual sexual relations; (6) HIV and AIDS; (7) sexual assault; (8) restriction of sexual interaction, and (9) staff training. The elements of this model policy are clear, comprehensive, and well written. However, some components (e.g., that every patient will receive a written copy of a policy with documentation of this in the clinical records) are overly prescriptive and may create their own difficulties. That said, interested readers who plan to develop a special policy should consult this important contribution. The chapter by Welch and Clements in this book also illustrates well how such a policy can be constructed and outlines the pragmatics of implementing a policy.

- clear definition of behaviors

- patient autonomy

- personal rights

- human sexuality and relationships

- contraception

- patient psychoeducation

- staff training

- explicit staff guidelines for dealing with consensual and non-consensual sex between patients

Figure 4.2. Important Components of Sexual Behavior Policy for a Psychiatric Facility.

Sexual Exploitation and Vulnerable Patients

The extent to which vulnerable patients can be protected from predatory sexual behavior by other patients is an important consideration. This is viewed by staff as a real concern (Civic et al., 1993) and is certainly a public concern (Mossman et al., 1997; Holbrook, 1989). In broad terms, patients who are most cognitively impaired and obviously lack competency to consent to sexual relations are at greatest risk for exploitation. This is particularly true for patients with comorbid mental retardation (Bhui & Puffett, 1994). Patients who are impulsive or those who are disinhibited as a consequence of either their psychosis or a mood disturbance are also at risk. The process of determining competency is described in detail elsewhere (see Noffsinger, this volume) and will not be repeated here. However, some comments are warranted on the broader impact of cognitive dysfunction in schizophrenia. Subtle cognitive impairment may be greater influence upon competency to consent to sex than for competency - standards, forced medication or forensic circumstances. It is now appreciated that cognitive impairment may be a prominent aspect of the illness for many patients and may be aggravated further by medication effects (Goldberg & Gold, 1995). It is now also appreciated that insight, a complex attribute of psychotic illness which exhibits a powerful influence upon behavior (Jones, 1995), is also intrinsically related to cognitive (particularly frontal lobe) dysfunction (Amador & Gorman, 1998). These considerations are important because they add further complexity to the assessment of sexual exploitation, freedom of expression, and autonomy in patients with serious mental illness (Coverdale et al., 1997; McCullough et al., 1992).

Management of Inhospital Sexual Incidents

An addition to the promulgation of hospital policies that guide staff response to sexual behavior among inpatients (see above), there are several clinical management procedures that should be addressed when inpatient sexual incidents occur. Some illustrative case vignettes of alleged inpatient sexual incidents are provided.

Case 1: A 41-year-old female with a diagnosis of schizophrenia and cocaine abuse alleged that she had been sexually molested. She stated that she awoke to find her night clothes in disarray and she suspected that "someone messed with me sexually". The nurse took a more detailed history and then reported the incident. The physician interviewed the patient and found no evidence of physical injury. The examination of the genital region was unremarkable. Other administrative staff were notified and the police conducted a thorough investigation. The claim of sexual molestation was unsubstantiated. No further incidents were recorded.

Case 2: A 41-year-old female with a diagnosis of schizophrenia alleged that a 39-year-old male patient with a diagnosis of schizophrenia had forced her to engage in oral sex. The allegation was not made until 10 days after the proposed incident. There were no witnesses to the incident and each patient gave conflicting information to the police. The investigation concluded that the claim was unsubstantiated.

Case 3: A 29-year-old female with a diagnosis of schizophrenia claimed that her breasts were fondled by a 29 year old male patient. The female pushed the patient away and reported the incident immediately to the staff. Both patients were interviewed by the physician. Administrative staff were also notified. The offending patient was transferred to another unit. The victim did not wish to pursue any further legal action. All events, notifications, and interventions were documented in the clinical records.

These vignettes describe alleged incidents of non-consensual sex and sexual activity occurring in the context of active psychosis. Accordingly, the immediate efforts were to stop the behavior and to protect the safety of the patients. In similar instances, symptom and behavior control may be achieved by counselling, staff redirection and by the appropriate use of medication. Seclusion or restraint of patients is not appropriate since it is punitive, reactive and humiliating. This option should be used only if the behavior escalates or continues to pose serious risk to other patients or staff. At the same time, it is important that the reasons for sexual impulsivity are thoroughly investigated. This investigation should begin, if at all possible, at the same time as management interventions are initiated. Delay in starting an investigation can result in an unclear picture because key details are forgotten by staff or patients. Additionally, fluctuation in the mental status of patients may complicate a delayed investigation. Finally, failure to retrieve key physical evidence (e.g., abrasions or analysis of bodily fluids) may be avoided through a prompt response.

At a minimum, each patient suspected of non-consensual sexual activity should be examined by a physician. This should occur in the context of detailed chart documentation of the incident, interventions and outcome. The hospital administration has a responsibility to conduct investigations in a thorough and efficient manner and to minimize bureaucratic delay. Decisions to proceed with legal charges are complex and are ultimately the responsibility of the victim and/or the hospital's chief executive officer. Hospital liability is minimized by an explicit policy, by clear staff directives, and by a consistent approach to the clinical management and administrative investigation of sexual incidents. It is important that predatory and nonconsensual sexual behavior be addressed by the treatment team. Staff should reemphasize the hospital policy and make explicit their concern for personal respect and for the protection of vulnerable patients. The patient's response and mental status should be documented in the clinical records. The team approach should be sensible, sensitive, and consistent with the hospital's policy (where one exists).

Contraception

Available literature (Carmen & Brady, 1996; Coverdale & Arouffo, 1989; also see chapters by Buckley *et al.*, McKinnon & Cournos) confirms that persons with serious mental illness use contraceptive techniques in an infrequent and inconsistent manner. Diclemente and Pointon (1993) reported that only 23% of patients who were sexually active used contraception on a consistent basis. In a recent outpatient study, Coverdale and colleagues (1997) reported a high rate of completed pregnancies among female patients (65%). They commented that this patient group is compromised by a failure of health authorities to provide comprehensive services regarding sexually transmitted diseases and family planning. This aspect of care is seldom emphasized and many mental health clinicians may be as uniformed as their patients regarding options for contraception. Contraceptive advice needs to be simple, accurate and delivered at a time when the patient can be receptive to this information (McEvoy *et al.*, 1983), i.e., contraception advice is unlikely to be helpful for the acutely psychotic patient who is just admitted to hospital. Information should be clear and given in vernacular terms. Also, whenever possible, information should be augmented by educational leaflets. Information should be shared in the context of a broader discussion of human sexuality, the desirability of pregnancy, and the patient's expectations (Lukoff *et al.*, 1986; also see Kopelwicz *et al.*, this volume).

A summary of the efficacy and pros and cons of each of the current form of contraception is given in Table 4.2. Techniques such as abstinence from sex, spermicide or gel applications are inherently unreliable even when practiced even by highly motivated couples. Therefore, these approaches are of as little benefit for persons with mental illness as they are for in the general population. Moreover, because of cognitive impairments and because hyperprolactinemia (from conventional antipsychotic medications) usually causes amenorrhoea, these methods should not be recommended as adequate contraception for persons with serious mental illness. This point is important to emphasize because female patients whose menstruation stops during treatment with conventional antipsychotic drugs may erroneously believe that these drugs also provide contraceptive protection. This is simply not the case. Newer antipsychotics are generally not associated with prolactin elevation and, consequently, are even less likely to impede contraception.

Barrier techniques (i.e., diaphragm, cervical cap, condoms) are acceptable and effective contraceptive options, particularly when used

Buckley *et al.*

Table 4.2. Comparative Efficacy and Acceptability of Current Forms of Contraception.

Method	Effect	Efficacy*	Strengths	Weaknesses
Abstinence techniques	timed to ovulation/ period of risk for contraception	20	natural; no health risks	limits sexual pattern; not reliable, especially for patients with menstrual disturbance to medications
Spermicide		21	no health risks; easy to apply	limits sexual pleasure; not reliable
Diaphragm, cervical cap	barrier to contraception	18	no health risks; inexpensive; enhanced efficacy when used with spermicide	may move and expose risk of conception may cause discomfort
Intrauterine Devise (IUD)	barrier to contraception	2	highly effective, reliable	needs health professional to insert; may cause discomfort, menorrhagia; may dislodge; potential for medical complications; needs periodic professional attention impedes
Condom	barrier to contraception	12 (5, with spermicide)	inexpensive; no health risk; effective with spermicide and with careful application	sexual pleasure;inadequate application tear exposes risk of conception

Table 4.2. (Continued)

Oral Contraceptive Pill (OCP)	disrupts ovulation pattern; induces 'hostile' cervical mucous	0.1 (0.5, progesterone only)	easy to use; widely acceptable; highly effective	not suitable for some; significant medical complications; may forget to take complete course of tablets
Depot Provera Injection	disrupts ovulation; produces 'hostile' cervical mucous	0.3	long lasting; reliable ensures compliance	major ethical obstacles; potential medical complications
Tubal Ligation	surgical blockage of fallopian ducts	0.4	long lasting; reliable	not popular; surgical procedure; risk of complications; may not be reversible if desired
Vasectomy	surgical blockage of vas deferens	0.1	long lasting; reliable	not popular; surgical procedure; risk of complications; may not be reversible if desired

* Expressed as percentage pregnancy rates during first year of careful use; no contraception is considered to be associated with an 85% pregnancy rate

in combination. However, ensuring adequate specialist follow-up and compliance are important. Condoms are notoriously apt to perforate. Condoms and spermicides in combination are a desirable option today because they are effective, relatively inexpensive, and they are also favored because they provide protection from HIV and other sexually transmitted diseases. However, inadequate and inconsistent use remain their major drawback. Persons with mental illness may engage in casual, unplanned sexual activity and forget or neglect to use condoms, just as frequently occurs in the general population.

The oral contraceptive pill (OCP) is the best current option to achieve contraceptive efficacy, reliability, and freedom of personal choice. The method of action of OCPs is not completely understood and varies according to the relative contributions of progesterone and estrogen derivatives. OCPs are thought to inhibit ovulation through the suppression of follicle stimulating hormone and luteinizing hormone, (i.e., gonadotrophin hormones that regulate ovulation and fertility). Combined OCPs (those containing both estrogen and progesterone) are thought to have additional effects by way of altering the cervical mucus to impede sperm penetration and by altering the receptiveness of the endometrium to implantation with a fertilized ovum. While widely used and prescribed, it is important to emphasize that OCPs are contraindicated for certain individuals. They are also associated with an elevated risk of significant morbidity in others. It should be appreciated that the lifestyle patterns of persons with serious mental illness (excessive smoking, obesity) and excess of physical comorbidity (cancer, cardiovascular illnesses) may significantly alter the risk-benefit ratio for OCP use. OCPs are generally contraindicated in the following circumstances: Thrombophlebitis; thromboembolic or ischemic cardiovascular disorders (particularly all forms of cerebral vascular disorder and coronary artery disease); breast, hepatic or endometrial carcinoma, or any estrogen dependent cancer; known or suspected pregnancy. They should also be used carefully in women who have other known risk factors for cardiovascular disorders (age, hypertension, lipid disorders, obesity, diabetes) or who have risk factors for neoplasia (family history or breast cancer, presence of breast modules or fibrocystic disease, abnormal mammogram, or cervical dysplasia). It is strongly recommended that OCPs be avoided for females who smoke since the relative risk of thromboembolic stroke for OCP users who also smoke (compared with non-smokers) is 7.6; this risk rises to 25.7 when females also have hypertension. In contrast, the risk of thromboembolic stroke for smokers who do not use OCP is 2.6. Overall, the risk of hemorrhage stroke and thromboembolic stroke in OCP users is between 2 and 10 times greater, respectively, than for those female who do not use the pill. This is an important consideration particularly given the high rates of smoking among patients with schizophrenia.

Table 4.3. Potential Drug Interactions Between the Oral Contraceptive Pill (OCP) and Psychotropic Medications.

Drug Class	Effect
Anticonvulsants, antidepressants, tricyclic antidepressants	OCPs reduce hepatic metabolism, side effects or toxicity of antidepressant medication may occur
Benzodiazepines	OCPs reduce hepatic metabolism; also glucuronidation may be impaired, leading to enhanced drug clearance
Beta Blockers	OCPs reduce hepatic metabolism
Phenytoin	Through induction of hepatic microsomal enzymes, may increase the metabolism of OCPs

Patients need to be given an adequate explanation of the risk factors and the procedure for effective contraception with OCPs. Clinicians should also be cognizant of drug-drug interactions that may occur between OCPs and various psychotropic medications. These interactions are highlighted in Table 4.3. It should not be assumed that consent or assent to OCPs use will translate into effective contraceptive practice since here again cognitive impairments may result in forgetfulness and neglect to complete the dosing schedule for the OCP. Additionally, compliance may be a factor much as it is for antipsychotic medication. This is particularly the case if OCP use has a coercive component and/or if the patient has a known history of poor medication compliance with psychotropic medications. Forced medroxyprogesterone injection (Depo Provera) is an alternative that can ensure compliance and contraception, but at the loss of personal autonomy. Methods of forced contraception are, therefore, less desirable and should only be considered as last resort. Forced contraception is fraught with complex legal and ethical concerns.

Abortion and Major Mental Illness

Females with psychosis who become pregnant may choose to abort. Additionally, abortion may be recommended by relatives or a guardian because of the female's incompetent mental status and inability to care for a child. The psychiatrist's duty here is to assess the female for competency to provide informed consent for decisions regarding the pregnancy and also to provide supportive counseling. However, the decision to abort or not extends well beyond the psychiatrist's involvement and is also beyond the institution's responsibility to provide patient care. Once competency has been established, the assessment and clinical decisions regarding abortion should be made by the patient in consultation with an obstetrician. In advance of any decision, the patient should have an expert assessment performed by the obstetrician.

Pregnancy and Mental Illness

Some females with known severe mental illness become pregnant (Miller and Finnerty, 1996). A very small minority of females develop major mental illness during pregnancy. In each circumstance, the overall risk of an unfavorable outcome is elevated, both for the mother and for the infant. However, the requirements of care differ between these two situations; broadly speaking, the management of the female with psychosis who becomes pregnant is more complex than that of the pregnant female who experiences psychotic symptoms of first onset during her pregnancy. The lack of comprehensive support services for persons with mental illness who become pregnant is glaring (see Deegan, this book).

Pregnancy is a perplexing and potentially fearful event for many women, irrespective of their level of mental stability. Counseling and supportive psychotherapy are therefore crucial to a successful pregnancy in a female with established psychosis. The mental health clinician must provide additional support that goes beyond routine, periodic outpatient review. The clinician must specifically explore and clarify the woman's expectations concerning her pregnancy. Reassurance must be given and the clinician needs to act as an educator, ensuring that the woman understands the stages of pregnancy, the anticipated changes, and the expectations that will be placed upon her by the obstetrician. The clinician has a duty to reemphasize in a supportive manner the guidelines set by the obstetrician. The importance of attending all obstetrician visits must be emphasized. The female should also be supported to attend these visits and to seek subsequent clarification from the mental health clinician if she does not understand any of the obstetrician's comments. Follow-up for all psychiatry visits is also essential. Compliance with psychotropic medication (if it is prescribed) is another critical issue. Unless the female is floridly psychotic when pregnancy is first determined, every effort should be made as early as possible in the pregnancy to discuss the risks and benefits of continued medication treatment. This discussion should occur in a manner and on a level of detail that is commensurate with the patient's capacity for insight. Relatives should also be informed and involved in the care, particularly since they may ultimately acquire guardianship for the infant if the female is unable to care for her baby.

Risks related to the female's psychotic illness are more significant for the pregnancy than any potential of teratogenicity from psychotropic medications. Psychosis that is inadequately managed contributes to the higher rates of obstetric and neonatal complications. Additionally, untreated or poorly controlled psychosis may expose the female to risk of self-harm and harm to the fetus. This may be either deliberate self-harm or inappropriate behavior (e.g., wandering, homelessness) consequent upon delusional thinking. The patient may be unable to appreciate the importance of pursuing a healthy lifestyle during the pregnancy. She may be reluctant to stop smoking and may miss or neglect appointments with her obstetrician. Her dietary habits may be unhealthy and she may lack the insight to comply with the obstetrician's request to take supplemental iron or vitamin tablets. Finally, persons with serious mental illness face social adversities such as inadequate housing, poor social support and financial strain. These factors of themselves mitigate against a healthy pregnancy. Accordingly, pregnancy in females with psychosis should be viewed as a high risk situation. This status should be evident to both the obstetrician and the psychiatrist. A mental status examination should be performed at every visit and changes in symptoms must be taken very seriously. Clinicians should question directly about suicidal and homicidal risk – it is a serious clinical misjudgement to underestimate the consequences of an inadequate risk.

It is important that every effort be made to establish a close collaboration between the obstetrician and the psychiatrist. Each possesses skills that complement the other's speciality. The mental health clinicians duties are to provide the obstetrician with a careful evaluation of the psychiatric risks in the pregnancy, of the female's risk of relapse, and the risk-benefit analysis of continued medication treatment.

A review of the potential deleterious impact of various psychotropic medications upon pregnancy and neonatal outcome is beyond the scope of this chapter. However, the relative risk for each agent is highlighted in Table 4.4. Also, the reader is referred to an excellent comprehensive review by Altshuler and colleagues on the use of psychotropic medications during pregnancy (Altshuler et al., 1996).

CONCLUDING REMARKS

Hospitals have potentially conflicting responsibility to protect patients and promote personal rights. The expression of human sexuality in hospitals exposes complex dilemmas which are best addressed by recognition of the 'real picture' and, accordingly, the implementation of policies and procedures that are meaningful. The distinction between acute care and long stay facilities is important in the determining the level of facilitation of sexual expression among inpatients. Fundamentally, issues of privacy, human respect, and personal

Table 4.4. Risks Associated with Psychotropic Drugs During Pregnancy.

Drug Class	Risk	Potential Adverse Effects
Antipsychotics	low	minor withdrawal effects in neonate; effects of novel antipsychotics are unknown
Tricylic Antidepressants	low	minor withdrawal effects in neonate
Selective Serotonin Reuptake Inhibitors	low-medium	recent study (Chambers *et al.*, 1996) suggests increased risk of minor anomalies, prematurity
Lithium	high	ebstein's cardiac anomaly upon exposure during first trimester; last trimester/puerperium exposure may cause lithium toxicity in neonate
Anticonvulsants	high	risk of cleft lip, spina bifida

fulfillment are the core constructs that should underlie the institution's policy on inpatient sex. Policies that are outdated, punitive in nature, or that fail to acknowledge these core constructs will be difficult to implement and, if so, they will expose the institution to the risk of medicolegal liability when sexual incidents occur.

REFERENCES

Akhtar, S. & Thompson, J.A. (1980). Schizophrenia and sexuality: a review and a report of twelve unusual cases — part I. *Journal of Clinical Psychiatry* 41(4):134–142.

Altshuler, L.L., Cohen, L., Szuba, M.P., Burt, V.K., Gitlin, M. & Mintz, J. (1996). Pharmacologic management of psychiatric illness during pregnancy: dilemmas and guidelines. *American Journal of Psychiatry* 153:592–606.

Anthony, W.A. (1993). Recovery from mental illness: The guiding vision of the mental health service system in the 1990s. *Psychosocial Rehabilitation Journal* 16(4):11–24.

Bachrach, L.L. (1996). The state of the state mental hospital in 1996. *Psychiatric Services* 47:1071–1078.

Bazel, D.I. (1995). Center for mental health law turning the corner: New ways to integrate mental health and substance abuse in the health care policy. Washington, DC, Author.

Bhui, K. & Puffel, A. (1994). Sexual problems in the psychiatric and mentally handicapped populations. *British Journal* 51(9):459–464.

Buckley, P.F. (1998). Novel antipsychotics and patient care in state hospitals. *Annals of Pharmacotherapy* 32:906–914.

Buckley, P.F. & Hyde, J.L. (1997). State hospital's responses to the sexual behavior of psychiatric inpatients. *Psychiatric Services* 48:398–399.

Carmen, E. & Brady, S.M. (1996). AIDS risk and prevention for the chronic mentally ill. *Hospital and Community Psychiatry* 41(6):652–657.

Chase, J.C. (1988). Sexual drive of patients in psychiatric hospitals. *British Medical Journal* 297:1129.

Civic, D., Walsh, G. & McBride, D. (1993). Staff perspectives on sexual behavior of patients in a state psychiatric hospital. *Hospital and Community Psychiatry* 44(9):887–889.

Cohen, D.D. & Tanenbaum, R.L. (1985). Sexuality education for staff in long-term psychiatric hospitals. *Hospital and Community Psychiatry* 36(2):187–189.

Cournos, F., Guido, J.R. & Coomaraswamy, S. *et al.* (1994). Sexual activity and risk of HIV infection among patients with schizophrenia. *American Journal of Psychiatry* 151(2):228–232.

Coverdale, J. & Arouffo, J. (1989). Family planning needs of female chronic psychiatric outpatients. *American Journal of Psychiatry* 146:1489–1491.

Coverdale, J.H., Bayer, T.L., McCullough, L.B. & Chervenak, F.A. (1993). Respecting the autonomy of chronic mentally ill women in decisions about contraception. *Hospital and Community Psychiatry* 44(7):671–674.

Coverdale, J.H., Turbott, S.H. & Roberts, H. (1997). Family planning needs and STD risk behaviors of female psychiatric outpatients. *British Journal of Psychiatry* 171:69–72.

Dalack, G.W. & Woodruff-Meador, J.H. (1996). Smoking, smoking withdrawal and schizophrenia: case reports and a review of the literature. *Schizophrenia Research* 133–141.

deLeon, J., Dadvand, M., Canuso, C., White, A.O., Stanilla, J.K. & Simpson, G.M. (1995). Schizophrenia and smoking: An epidemiological survey in a state hospital. *American Journal of Psychiatry* 152:453–455.

Diclemente, R.J. & Ponton, L.E. (1993). HIV-related risk behaviors among psychiatrically hospitalized adolescents and school-based adolescents. *American Journal of Psychiatry* 150:324–325.

Goldberg, T.E. & Gold, J.M. (1995). Neurocognitive deficits in schizophrenia. In schizophrenia, Hirsch, S.R., Weinberger, D.W., (eds.). Blackwell Science LTD, Oxford, England.

Grassi, L. (1996). Risk of HIV infection in psychiatrically ill patients. *AIDS CARE* 8(1):103–116.

Grunebaum, H. & Abernethy, V. (1975) Ethical issues in family planning for hospitalized psychiatric patients. *American Journal of Psychiatry* 132:236–240.

Hogan, M. (1996) State Mental Health Systems: Their Evolution and Use of Economic Tools. In Moscarelli, M., Rupp, A. & Sartorius, N. (eds.): *Handbook of Mental Health Economics and Health Policy* Volume I, Schizophrenia, New York: John Wiley and Sons. (pp. 515–524).

Holbrook, T. (1989). Policing sexuality in a modern state hospital. *Hospital and Community Psychiatry* 40(1):75–79.

Imbornoni, S., Donenwirth, K., Orr, B., Hagesfeld, T., Gintoli, G. & Buckley, P.F. (1997) Objective measurement of psychiatric symptoms: A quality improvement process for inpatient care. *Joint Commission Journal on Quality Improvement* 23:183–195.

Johnson, A.M., Wadsworth, J. & Wellings, K. *et al.* (1992). Sexual lifestyles and HIV risk. *Nature* 360:410–412.

Jones, G.H. (1995). Informed consent in chronic schizophrenia? *British Journal of Psychiatry* 167:565–568.

Keitner, G. & Grof, P. (1981) Sexual and emotional intimacy between psychiatric inpatients: Formulating a policy. *Hospital and Community Psychiatry* 32(3):188–193.

Lukoff, D., Sullivan, J.G. & Goisman, R.M. (1992). Sex and AIDS education. Liberman, R.P., Goldstein, A.P., Krasner, L. (eds.). Boston: Allyn and Bacon, 171–182.

McCullough, L.B., Coverdale, J.H., Bayer, T. *et al.* (1992). Ethically justified guidelines for family planning interventions to prevent pregnancy with female chronically mentally ill patients. *American Journal of Obstetrics and Gynecology* 167:19–25.

McEvoy, J.P., Hatcher, A., Applebaum, P.S. & Abernethy, V. (1983). Chronic schizophrenic women's attitudes toward sex, pregnancy, birth control, and childbearing. *Hospital and Community Psychiatry* 34:536–539.

Miller, L.J. & Finnerty, M. (1996). Sexuality, pregnancy and childbearing among women with schizophrenia – spectrum disorders. *Psychiatric Services* 47:502–506.

Mossman, D., Perlin, M.L. & Dorfman, D.A. (1997). Sex on the wards: connundra for clinicians. *Academy of Psychiatry and the Law* 25:441–460.

Vandereycken, W. (1993) Shrinking sexuality: The half-known sex life of psychiatric patients. *Therapeutic Communities* 14(3):143–149.

Welch, S. & Clement, J. (1996) Devising a policy for inpatient sex. *Canadian Journal of Psychiatry* 41:273–276.

Welch, S., Meagher, J., Soos, J. & Bhopal, J. (1991) Sexual behavior of hospitalized chronic psychiatric patients. *Hospital and Community Psychiatry* 42(8):855–856.

5

Developing and Implementing a Policy for Consensual Sex Between Inpatients

STEVEN J. WELCH, GERRIT W. CLEMENTS and MARGARET E. MOREAU

Riverview Hospital is British Columbia's (B.C.) tertiary care psychiatric hospital. It is a university-affiliated teaching hospital with full accreditation from the Canadian Council on Health Services Accreditation. The Specialized Rehabilitation Program (SRP) (referred to as the Continuing Treatment Program in prior publications) at the hospital cares for approximately 260 patients with chronic psychiatric disorders, primarily schizophrenia (66%), schizoaffective disorder (12%), and bipolar disorder (8%), who have not responded to treatment in community hospitals or residences. The average number of years current patients have been in the SRP, inclusive of all admissions, is 7.5. The majority of patients are male (58.9%). Patients' average age is 39.2 years.

The policy on patient sexuality described below was created specifically for SRP patients and initially implemented on a pilot basis on SRP wards. Although the policy recently was extended to other programs within Riverview Hospital, the discussion that follows will pertain to the SRP experience.

The purpose of this chapter is to familiarize the reader with the Riverview Hospital Policy on Patient Sexuality and to discuss problems encountered with its development and implementation. Solutions to the problems encountered are suggested.

RIVERVIEW HOSPITAL POLICY ON PATIENT SEXUALITY

A detailed description of the Riverview Hospital Policy on Patient Sexuality is available elsewhere (Welch & Clements, 1996). A brief description follows.

The policy addresses a number of specific aspects of the more global topic of patient sexuality. The first part of the policy outlines the rights of patients and duties of hospital administrative and clinical staff, according to legal opinion. The spirit of each right and duty stems from the *Canadian Charter of Rights and Freedoms* (1982), provincial legislation, the common law, and the *Riverview Hospital Charter of Patient Rights* (1994). A copy of the *Charter of Patient Rights* may be obtained from the hospital.

In summary, both involuntary and voluntary long stay hospitalized psychiatric patients have a right to sexual intimacy in a private and dignified setting. Staff have a duty to accept and address patients' sexuality, regardless of sexual orientation or marital status, in an empathic, nonjudgmental, and humane manner. The hospital administration has a duty to take reasonable care to protect patients from possible harm arising from sexual encounters and to provide education and rehabilitation relevant to patient sexuality. Although the policy has not been tested through litigation in Canada, it has been accepted by the Ombudsman for the Province of B.C. (1994) and by the Canadian Council on Health Facilities Accreditation (1994). Moreover, the premises of the policy are consistent with opinions expressed in a Working Paper on sexual activity among institutionalized persons sponsored by the McGill Centre for Medicine, Ethics and Law (McSherry & Somerville, 1996).

The Riverview Hospital Policy on Patient Sexuality attempts to balance patient rights and hospital duties in a reasonable manner. Such balance was a guiding principle in creating the policy. Consequently, conditions were placed on patients' rights when needed as a reasonable means of protecting patients from harm. These conditions will be apparent to the reader as other components of the policy are summarized below.

The second part of the policy outlines the environmental, educational, and therapeutic supports that are to be available to patients. Thus this part of the policy specifies the infrastructure necessary within the hospital in order for policy implementation to be viable. In brief, the policy calls for: (1) privacy curtains around dormitory beds, removable for certain clinical reasons; (2) private suites for purposes of sexual intimacy, accessible if certain conditions are met; (3) free condom availability, usually via machines in washrooms; (4) a sex education course available on a regular basis; (5) counseling, when requested, for sexual abuse, sexual dysfunction, sexually transmitted diseases, birth control and abortion. Additionally, education regarding the policy and patient sexuality are mandatory for clinical staff.

The third part of the policy outlines the orientation, assessment, and treatment protocol to be followed when a patient is admitted to a hospital program. The patient is to be informed about the policy, a sexual history is to be taken, the patient is to be asked about his or her desire for birth control, testing for sexually transmitted diseases, or counseling regarding any sexual issue, and the patient is encouraged to attend the sex education course. A modified version of the Sexual History/HIV Risk Assessment questionnaire (Brady & Carmen, 1990) is used to facilitate the acquisition of this information.

The fourth part of the policy deals exclusively with masturbation because this is a common form of sexual expression within the hospital, because it sometimes occurs in inappropriate places, and because it is a relatively safe form of sexual behavior (Welch & Clements, 1996). The policy states that a physician or nurse is to inform each patient that masturbation is acceptable within the confines of their privacy curtain. Patients are to be allowed to possess erotic pictures or literature provided that the material is legally available and on the condition that it is not considered to be countertherapeutic for any specific patient. Each bed area is to contain tissues and a waste basket.

The fifth part of the policy deals with patient access to private suites located in a cottage on the hospital grounds for the purpose of sexual intimacy. The number of days per week the cottage is open depends upon patient demand. Consistent with the duty to protect, the cottage displays posters and literature on prevention of sexually transmitted diseases, and each suite contains condoms and an alarm button connected to a staff office on a different floor. A Cottage Supervisor is always in the cottage when patients are in the suites. The Cottage Supervisor, who is a psychiatric nurse, receives information from wards about which patients are eligible to use the suites, accepts reservations from eligible patients, and informally assesses each patient for problems such as decompensation or intoxication before permitting access to the suites.

Consistent with the intention of balancing patients' rights with the hospital's duty to protect, the policy requires that certain conditions be met and documented on a form entitled "Application for Use of Private Suite" before a patient is allowed access to a private suite. The policy states: (1) a patient must complete the sex education course; (2) a patient's subsequent request to use a suite shall be granted unless there is a known medical or psychiatric contraindication (the former being a physical condition that would make sexual activity dangerous to the patient or partner, such as HIV infection; the latter being a mental condition that renders the patient incapable of consenting or behaving responsibly); (3) a patient is to be presumed capable of consensual and responsible sex unless explicit indicators of possible incapability are present; (4) if indicators of incapability are present, a test of capability is to be applied; (5) if a patient is found incapable, the patient's treatment plan must be reviewed and changes made that may help make the patient capable; (6) patients found incapable may reapply in one month, and after three successive denials may appeal to an independent psychiatrist; and (7) patients granted access to the private suites may have that access suspended or revoked via a physician's order, should indicators of possible incapability arise.

In B.C. the presumption of capability to make and act on one's own decisions (item 3 above) follows from the common law and is expressly set out in recently enacted adult guardianship legislation (*Adult Guardianship Act*). Capability must be assumed unless and until a clear indicator of possible incapability is present. A checklist of indicators of possible incapability was created from suggestions in the literature (Alexander, 1988; Freedman, Stuss & Gordon, 1991) to help treatment team members make this judgement.

No test of capability (item 4 above) to consent to sexual intimacy or engage in safe sex was available for use as a model. Consequently, a three part test was developed based on the general common law test of understanding the nature and consequences of one's decisions and actions. The first part is a mental status exam designed to detect a disorder of attention, memory, language, thought, perception, mood or control severe enough to render the patient incapable in one or both of these two areas. This requires a clinical judgment. The second part requires the patient to demonstrate a factual understanding of the meaning of certain relevant terms (e.g., "safe sex"). The third part requires the patient to demonstrate a more pragmatic understanding of relevant issues and the risks of engaging in sexual behavior (e.g., "How do you use a condom?"; "What will happen to you if you get AIDS?"). All information required to answer these questions is presented in the sex education course.

REASONS FOR DEVELOPING THE POLICY

The need for formal hospital policies regarding patient sexuality has been recognized for some time. Nevertheless, there are so few reports of such policies in the professional literature as to force the conclusion that they are almost nonexistent (Firn, 1994; Keitner & Grof, 1981; Welch & Clements, 1996). This is most unfortunate because there are numerous reasons why every psychiatric hospital should have a written policy on patient sexuality.

First, there is no question that some hospitalized psychiatric patients are sexually active (Bell, Wringer, Davidhizar & Samuels, 1993; Cournos *et al.*, 1994; Welch & Clements, 1996). Consequently, if our contention that patients have a right to sexual intimacy in a humane and dignified setting is correct (Welch & Clements, 1996), a formal policy likely will be required to ensure that such a setting is available.

Second, chronic mental disorder is now recognized as an HIV risk factor (Gottesman & Groome, 1997). The relationship between HIV and serious mental illness is reviewed by McKinnon and colleagues in this volume and consequently will not be discussed further here. If our contentions that patients have a right to sexual intimacy and that hospital administration and staff have a duty to take reasonable care to protect patients from harm arising from sexual encounters (Welch & Clements, 1996) are correct, then a written policy is essential to provide staff with guidelines for protecting patients from harm. Parenthetically, even if a duty to protect did not exist in law, it would certainly exist in professional ethics.

Third, the data available suggest that HIV seroprevalence is higher in psychiatric inpatients than in the general population (Volavka *et al.*, 1992). Once again, see McKinnon and colleagues in this volume for greater detail. Administrators of hospitals for persons with chronic mental illness should expect the number of HIV infected patients to increase, and there is some evidence that this is occurring (Cournos, Empfield, Horwath & Kramer, 1986). Whether the duty to protect is based in law or professional ethics, it is very clear that hospital administration and clinical staff must take action immediately to attempt to counter the risk to patients. As we have argued (Welch & Clements, 1996) a written policy specifying reasonable means of reducing the risk of HIV infection is far more likely to be effective than leaving staff to deal with this issue on their own.

Fourth, many chronic psychiatric patients have difficulty establishing intimate relationships, show a high rate of sexual dysfunction, and engage in sexual behaviors that may be disturbing to others or dangerous to themselves or others (Welch & Clements, 1996). This topic is addressed more fully by Kopelwitz and colleagues in this volume. If our contention that psychiatric hospitals have a duty to provide education and rehabilitation pertaining to patient sexuality (Welch & Clements, 1996) is correct, it is likely that a written policy will be required to ensure that these problems are assessed and treated.

Fifth, there is some evidence that patients with psychiatric disorders have a higher prevalence of sexual abuse in childhood than do nonpatient samples (Goodman, Rosenberg, Mueser & Drake, 1997). See Rosenberg and colleagues in this volume for more information. Since there is no reason to believe that the sequelae of sexual abuse in chronic psychiatric inpatients would be any less severe than in the general population (Jacobson & Herald, 1990), assessment and counseling should be available to these patients. This is most likely to occur within the context of a written policy.

Sixth, although clinicians became aware of the substantial adverse effects of psychotropic drugs soon after their introduction in the 1950's on patients' sex lives, these side effects tend to be underestimated or ignored in clinical practice (Vandereycken, 1993). This topic is addressed in detail by Millner and colleagues and by Deegan in this volume. In consideration of the fact that medication-induced sexual dysfunction may reduce patient compliance with medication

(Fleischhacker, Meise, Gunther & Kurz, 1994) and that treatment of medication-induced sexual dysfunction may be effective (Gitlin, 1994), clinicians should routinely ask patients about their sexual functioning. Since many clinicians appear to be reluctant to discuss this issue (Vandereycken, 1993), a formal policy requiring a routine evaluation of patients' sexual functioning is important.

Seventh, nurses and other clinical staff have a variety of concerns regarding patient sexuality. These include confusion about how to respond to patients' sexual needs and behavior; how to prevent pregnancy and STDs; whether or not to provide patients with increased privacy and if so, how; whether sexual education or activity will exacerbate mental illness; patient ability to consent and possible victimization of patients; sexual bartering; absence of clear policies to guide decision making; feeling uncomfortable discussing sexual issues; and what to do when the personal values of individual staff conflict with patient desires and values (Civic *et al.*, 1993; Davidhizar, Boonstra, Lutz & Poston, 1991; Woolf & Jackson, 1996). A formal policy on patient sexuality could and should address all these concerns. Having questions answered usually helps to alleviate anxiety to some degree.

Eighth, although some staff fear that they may be held legally liable if they permit patients to be sexually intimate and some harm then befalls one or both patients (e.g., pregnancy, contraction of an STD), or family members become distraught (Commons, Bohn, Godon, Hauser & Gutheil, 1992; Perlin, 1993; Walker & Fraiser, 1994), we (Welch & Clements, 1996) have argued that a formal written policy is more likely to reduce the potential for liability and thereby protect staff. The reason is directly related to the reasons for developing a policy reviewed above. Administrative and clinical staff know, or ought to know, that some chronic psychiatric patients are sexually active, at substantial risk for contracting HIV, and have a variety of sexual problems. Consequently, failure to develop a policy to address these issues could be seen as a neglect of moral responsibility and noncompliance with a legal duty. The presence of a policy that makes a reasonable effort to balance patient rights to sexual intimacy in a dignified setting with the hospital's duty to protect patients from harm protects staff by taking guesswork and personal opinions out of the decision-making process. Failure to develop a policy leaves staff uncertain about how to deal with sexual issues and increases the risk of staff believing that either they need not address these issues or of decisions about sexual behavior being made on the basis of idiosyncratic value systems (Cohen & Tanenbaum, 1985; Firn, 1994; Holbrook, 1989).

POLICY DEVELOPMENT: PROBLEMS AND SOLUTIONS

In response to both patient concerns regarding their sexual needs and staff concerns regarding the sexual behavior of some patients, the Program Director of the SRP requested the SRP Multidisciplinary Committee to form a task force on patient sexuality. After assessing the sexual needs of patients in the SRP (see Welch & Clements, 1996), the primary job of the task force became policy development and implementation.

The task force solicited representation from as many relevant stakeholders as possible. This included representatives from clinical departments such as medicine, nursing, pastoral care, psychology and social work, as well as from administrative and related committees such as the Ethics Committee, Health Education Services, and the Patient Environmental Needs Committee. Additionally, representatives were solicited from patients through the hospital's Patient Empowerment Society (PES) and from family members through the Riverview Hospital Family Group. Representation from a special interest group external to the hospital, the B.C. Schizophrenia Society, also was obtained. Legal representation was obtained from the Mental Health Law Program at the hospital and from the B.C. Ministry of Health Special Health Law Consultant.

Fear of Legal Liability

It was anticipated that a task force with so many representatives would slow the process of policy development but it seemed likely that each stakeholder group would have unique concerns that would be best identified at the outset. The inclusion of all stakeholders in the process of policy development is essential, even though it slows the process, because management of patient sexuality is an emotionally laden issue and stakeholder groups from patients and staff to administration and parents will want to feel that they have had some say in the process in order to reduce their personal concerns and anxieties.

As expected, the varied representation resulted in a wide range of opinions and concerns. In general, the patient representatives were relatively liberal in their views. While recognizing the need to protect fellow patients from harm, they were in favor of minimizing the required safeguards for fear that many patients would not attempt to gain access to the private suite if there were too many preconditions. In contrast, clinical staff representatives and family representatives were more conservative and lobbied for a number of safeguards to fulfil the hospital's duty to protect. While each of these stakeholder groups tended to have different concerns, the fear of legal liability was prominent for all but the patients. This fear of possible litigation became problematic in that clinical and family representatives and their stakeholder groups became quite preoccupied with the issue. Not only did this preoccupation slow the work of the task force but also resulted in our failure to fully attend to the PES representatives who were less concerned with the legalities and more concerned with the practicalities of the policy. The outcome was a policy that is fairly conservative in terms of the duty to protect and not as patient-friendly as it could be. This issue will be discussed in more detail later in the chapter.

Regarding a solution to this problem, which Brodsky (1988) has referred to as "litigaphobia" (p. 497), we suggest that policy developers who are clinical staff or family members but not lawyers be prepared to seek and accept the advice of legal consultants rather than engage in the folly of legal speculation. Also, bear in mind that a literature exists which suggests that physicians and mental health professionals significantly overestimate the risk of being sued (Brodsky, 1988; Lawthers et al., 1992). Moreover, it is simply intolerable for fear of liability to impede actions which are otherwise reasonable and ethically justified. Finally, remember our contention that the presence of a reasonable policy is likely to reduce legal liability even if the policy is not perfect (Welch & Clements, 1996).

Representation of Stakeholders

Because the task force worked from a consensus model and therefore felt obliged to accommodate the concerns of all its members, discussions about many aspects of the policy were lengthy and often did not lead to decisions that were satisfactory to all. This in itself is to be expected because, with a large number of stakeholder groups involved, negotiation and compromise are inevitable. The problem encountered was not the diversity of opinion or the requirement for negotiation and compromise. Rather, there was a problem because we had failed to ensure that each stakeholder group was prepared to accept the outcome agreed to by its representative(s). That is, even after hours of discussion led to resolution of an issue within the task force, members of stakeholder groups external to the task force did not feel bound to accept what their representative(s) had agreed to. Consequently, the same issues were sent back to the task force numerous times, making it very difficult to resolve many details of the policy.

A solution to this problem must involve having stakeholder groups agree, a priori, to abide by the outcomes negotiated by their representatives. To facilitate this, stakeholder groups should try to identify their major concerns before the process of policy development begins. They should elect a representative whom they trust to present their concerns during policy development. Most important, they must realize that different stakeholder groups will have different concerns and they must be prepared to accept whatever compromise position their representative finds reasonable and agrees to.

POLICY IMPLEMENTATION: PROBLEMS AND SOLUTIONS

Hospital administration realized the need for a policy on patient sexuality and the draft version prepared by the task force was approved by all administrative levels with few modifications. The fact that the task force had representation from virtually all stakeholder groups who otherwise might have objected to the policy, that legal opinion had been solicited, and that the policy was quite conservative in terms of the duty to protect, likely alleviated many administrative concerns and facilitated administrative acceptance. The task force was given authority to implement the policy in the SRP on a pilot basis. Implementation proved to be a lengthy process fraught with difficulties. The major problems encountered are addressed in the following sections.

Preparing Clinical Staff

The task force realized that staff education about the sexuality policy and adequate preparation regarding their role in its implementation was essential to gain the support of clinical staff. At one of the early task force meetings one nursing representative astutely reported that, "Preparing the staff in a careful, sensitive, and thorough manner is of the utmost importance for unless staff embrace the policy and work towards its implementation, the enterprise will surely fail." Initially one-day workshops were planned for the nurses and health care workers on each of the pilot wards. However, senior clinical administration decided to reduce the sessions from one day to 90 minutes due to budgetary constraints. Although 91% of the staff who attended the education sessions indicated that the time allotted for education was "just right," the spectrum of comments provided on evaluation forms demonstrated that many staff remained unconvinced of the value or feasibility of the policy. While some staff commented favorably on the policy, concerns were raised about moral and legal implications, and some strong negative opinions were expressed. During education sessions staff also raised questions that appeared to reflect a good deal of underlying anxiety about sexuality in general and legal liability in particular. They wondered if providing a privacy suite was advocating sexual contact, if promiscuous patients should have access to the suite, if capable patients would be allowed to engage in extramarital sex, if conception could result in a lawsuit, and if there would be reprisals against staff who chose, for moral reasons, not to follow the policy. Answers to all these questions had been provided but apparently not heard by all.

Since the introduction of the sexuality policy, a vocal minority of staff have continued to maintain that they are unwilling to deal with patients' sexual issues. The level of resistance and anxiety in some clinical staff also resulted in jokes and name-calling directed at the Cottage Supervisor. Needless to say, the minority negative opinion of these staff about the policy, and skepticism about its value, significantly hampered implementation. We strongly suspect that the vocal minority inhibited staff who were supportive of the policy.

Resistance to addressing patient sexuality is not unique to Riverview Hospital. Many researchers have commented on the tendency for some clinical staff to be quite biased against the idea of providing privacy suites or even sex education to patients. Wasow (1980) interviewed health care personnel regarding a room for privacy. Twenty-three of 38 staff were in favor while 15 were against the idea. Of those opposed, most were nurses. As occurred at Riverview, some of the minority were quite vocal about their opposition. Wasow (1980) indicated that a primary goal for inservice staff training would need to include increasing staff comfort levels about sexuality and increasing tolerance of patient needs. Thus, overcoming sources of staff resistance was seen as an essential first step in the introduction of any program related to patient sexuality. Trudel and Disjardins (1992) reviewed a number of studies related to staff attitudes regarding patient sexuality. They concluded that policies on sexuality are necessary but also note that nurses appear to be less tolerant of propositions such as making private rooms available to patients than are other types of mental health workers. In view of this finding, they caution that the implementation of a policy on sexuality cannot occur without relevant staff collaboration. Davidhizar et al. (1991) also report an experience similar to Riverview's. In developing a program on safer sex for psychiatric inpatients, they found that some staff made frequent derogatory comments and sexual jokes. Some staff refused to hand out condoms because it was against their religion. Staff were described as generally uncomfortable with the subject of patient sexuality. The authors point out that the support of staff is essential to the success of a program and that staff bias against sex education or accepting patients as sexual individuals must be addressed before staff support can develop. Experiences of staff resistance have also been reported by others who have usually concluded that it is necessary to invest time in preparing staff to help them overcome their anxieties and bias (Cohen & Tanenbaum, 1985; Leichtman, 1990; Shaul & Morrey, 1980; Wolf & Menninger, 1973; Woolf & Jackson, 1996).

As indicated above, nurses appear to be among the most resistant of clinical staff to sexuality policies. In fairness to nurses, this may be because they are the staff who are most often exposed to patient sexual behavior and most often required to respond to it (Trudel & Desjardins, 1992; Wasow, 1980). For example, Akhtar, Crocker, Dickey, Helfrich & Rheuban (1977) found that when inpatients were discovered engaging in some form of sexual behavior, 91% of these discoveries were made by a nurse. The point here is not to be unduly critical of nurses but only to note that, as the clinical staff most likely to be confronted by patient sexual behavior, it is of paramount importance that nurses in particular receive the necessary preparation before any attempt is made to implement a sexuality policy. To underscore this point, Bor and Watts (1993) have noted that emerging medical and social problems such as HIV infection will result in increasing pressure on nurses to become skilled in discussing sexual issues with patients. Consistent with this contention, Civic et al. (1993) found that 83.7% of a sample of psychiatric staff consisting primarily of nurses and aides stated that they needed more training in communication skills and in responding to situations involving patient sexual behavior. The only training need rated by this sample as more important related to learning more about HIV and other sexually transmitted disease.

While the foregoing makes the problems we encountered at Riverview quite clear, the solution is less so. Because the nurses and health care workers in our pilot program received only 90 minutes of education about the policy and their role in its implementation, it is reasonable to speculate that this was simply insufficient time to adequately address staff concerns and anxieties, leaving residual bias and resistance in some staff. A brief review of the available literature is consistent with this hypothesis. Leichtman (1990) reported that 20 staff who were to provide sex education to hospitalized patients received eight 90-minute training sessions. This author stated that after this relatively extensive training, "There was little doubt that the hospital was ready for a sex education program for patients... By this point, sex education had become an established part of hospital treatment rather than a threatening intrusion" (p. 46–47). Cohen and Tanenbaum (1985) provided sexuality education for 32 staff of four long-term psychiatric hospitals in the form of six 2 1/2-hour sessions. Follow-up sessions occurred in three of the four hospitals. Outcome was not clearly described but three of the hospitals later formed task forces composed in part of the original program participants. These task forces apparently arranged additional training activities for other hospital staff. The reader is left with the impression that resistance was minimal. Shaul and Morrey (1980) provided two series of four 90-minute sessions on sexuality to 40 staff of a state mental hospital. Few staff were able to attend all four sessions because funding for coverage on their wards was not available. However, staff evaluations of the sessions were described as quite positive. No mention was made of any remaining resistance. Wolfe and Menninger (1973) provided seminars on human sexuality to 10 staff by way of six 90-minute sessions. They reported, "The seminars helped reduce anxiety about human sexuality and enabled staff to deal more comfortably with sexual problems on the ward" (p. 147). These studies strongly imply that adequate preparation of clinical staff prior to policy implementation is associated with success. The parameters of "adequate preparation" are not entirely clear, but the studies reviewed above suggest that the 90-minute session offered at Riverview should have been increased to four 90-minute sessions, at minimum.

The literature also makes clear that staff preparation must provide more than knowledge about the policy; it also must reduce staff anxiety and increase comfort levels with regard to patient sexuality. It is necessary to provide enough time for facilitators to promote discussion among staff of the variety of concerns they have. In addition, more specific strategic interventions may be helpful. For example, Withersty (1976) used a behavioral technique known as behavior rehearsal to help both desensitize nurses with regard to anxiety caused by patient sexual behavior and to provide them with appropriate coping strategies. A male psychology intern played the role of a patient and presented staff with realistic problems related to sexuality. Staff role-played their responses to these problems, often receiving suggestions from other staff who watched. Thus the staff were repeatedly exposed to situations they initially found anxiety-inducing and they learned a repertoire of desirable responses to those situations which replaced their original tendency to avoid the situations. The author reports that the behavior rehearsal was well received and that participants indicated that their anxiety levels decreased.

Keitner and Grof (1981) have suggested that staff anxiety related to patient sexuality will be decreased if the team psychiatrist takes a leadership role when addressing sexual issues. Psychiatrists who take a passive or unclear approach to patient sexuality leave other members of the team to respond in their own idiosyncratic and probably contradictory ways, leading to an increase in anxiety. Unfortunately, physicians tend to be as uncomfortable with patient sexuality as many other staff, and they tend to harbor inaccurate beliefs such as the pervasive idea that patient sexual activity may retard recovery or that appearing to sanction patient sex will result in their being sued (Bhui & Puffett, 1994; Keitner & Grof, 1981; Walker & Fraiser, 1994; Wolfe & Menniger, 1973; Woolf & Jackson, 1996). It is reasonable to assume that physicians, like other staff, will need adequate preparation to enhance their comfort level with a policy on patient sexuality. Physicians at Riverview were provided with a one-hour education session about the policy. Undoubtedly this was insufficient time, as was the case with the nurses.

In retrospect, our failure to adequately prepare clinical staff for the policy and their role in it was not due to a lack of awareness within the task force of the importance of adequate preparation. It was due more to difficulty in obtaining the strong and sustained directive from senior clinical administrators needed to permit a greater degree of preparation. Of course fiscal constraints played a role too. Davidhizar et al. (1991) have noted that administrative commitment is essential to implementing a program on sexuality in a psychiatric hospital. Administrators must be seen to be in firm support of the program, must give strong directives when necessary, and must ensure that sufficient time and resources are available for adequate staff preparation.

Preparing Family Members

Preparing family members for the policy was not quite as problematic as preparing clinical staff. The members of the Riverview Family Group initially were very concerned about the sexuality policy. They had four major worries. First, they felt that it might increase the vulnerability of hospital patients to exploitation and abuse. Second, they voiced concerns about the ability of two patients to parent a child, should a pregnancy occur, and they were fearful that the family of the ill sons or daughters who produced a child would feel a responsibility to raise the grandchild who, unfortunately, might be genetically predisposed to develop the same illness as the son or daughter. Third, they wondered whether the hospital would be legally liable if some harm befell a patient due to the policy, and they requested that the hospital seek legal advice on this point. Fourth, the impact of B.C.'s new *Adult Guardianship Act* was raised. This legislation, when implemented, will provide for substitute decision-makers if a patient is found unable to make his or her own decisions. A family member wondered if, in the case where the Office of the Public Trustee held "committee of person" for a patient, the Public Trustee would have to be asked if the patient could use the private suite.

Fortunately we were able to address all four concerns to the satisfaction of the family representatives on the task force and most members of the Riverview Family Group. Regarding the issue of vulnerability and abuse, family members were able to see that a policy that provided education, examined a patient's capability to consent, and provided a safe and supervised environment for sexual intimacy should reduce the potential for exploitation and abuse. The concern that two patients might produce a child was addressed in several ways. Parent group members agreed that the sex education, assessment of birth control needs, and provision of condoms, all required by the policy, should reduce the likelihood of an unplanned pregnancy. The case of an individual or couple who might want to conceive was addressed in the following manner, at the suggestion of the family representatives. First, the basic sex education curriculum included a brief and simplified account of the genetics of mental illness to ensure that patients knew that they had an increased risk of producing a child with mental illness. Second, a question testing this knowledge was added to the test of capability. Because these solutions originated with the parent group, it is not surprising that they were happy with them. Third, to address the concerns of legal liability, the parent group requested that legal advisors be added to the task force and they were. Parents were able to accept the lawyers' contention that a policy on patient sexuality would focus attention on the hospital's duty to protect the patients and reduce the potential for litigation. Regarding the fourth concern, the lawyers on the task force doubted that the authority of a committee of person extended to decision-making regarding sexual matters. Nevertheless, the Office of the Public Trustee was asked for an opinion. The Public Trustee examined the policy and concluded that it contained reasonable safeguards to protect patients from harm. The Public Trustee did not feel the need to be contacted if a patient for whom the Public Trustee held committeeship of person was granted access to the private suite.

Finally, medical and psychological representatives on the task force attended the Family Group on several occasions to discuss the policy and answer questions. Apparently these combined actions alleviated the anxiety of many family members. Eventually the Riverview Family Group commended the task force for "taking up an extremely difficult job of implementing this new and important service to the hospital."

Preparing Patients

A survey had indicated that almost 50% of SRP patients had engaged in some form of sexual activity during the past year and that over 40% of the patients wanted a more private place for sexual activity (Welch & Clements, 1996). Consequently, our expectation was that patients would be interested in obtaining information about the new Policy on Patient Sexuality. A number of vehicles were used to inform patients about the policy.

The Chairperson of the Patient Empowerment Society (PES) was a member of the task force during the creation and implementation of the policy, and a number of patients had served as representatives to the task force as well. The PES held its own meetings on a regular basis and thus served as a conduit of information about the policy to the patient population. Additionally, a patient information session was held at a clubhouse on the hospital grounds. An open house for patients was held at the cottage containing the privacy suites. Patients also were informed of the policy at least once at community meetings held on each ward. Copies of the policy were available on each ward for perusal by the patients and brochures that gave a brief description of the policy were handed out. The sex education course and availability of the privacy suites were well publicized in the manner described above.

Approximately one-third of the patients on the pilot wards expressed an interest in attending the sex education course. However, only a small number actually came to the course. Sixteen months after the sex education course was initiated, only 33 patients had participated in the course. During the first year only one couple used the privacy suite, although other patients were granted access to the suite but ultimately did not use it for various reasons (e.g., discharge from hospital; partner not eligible to use suite).

Although informal data indicated that a number of patients were still engaging in sexual activity in hospital buildings or on the grounds, fewer patients than anticipated attended the sex education course or used the privacy suites. This is a problem because uninformed patients using stairwells and grounds for sexual activity are at increased risk for becoming pregnant and contracting HIV. There are several possible reasons why patients have not taken advantage of the sex education course or privacy suites, which we now discuss.

Although they were informed about the policy as described above, it may be that patients with serious mental illness require multiple prompts or reminders. Patients with schizophrenia have specific neurological and cognitive deficits which may lead to inaction despite the intention of engaging in a behavior. For example, there is considerable evidence that frontal lobe dysfunction is present in at least some forms of schizophrenia (Nasrallah, 1992). Thus a patient with the intention of taking a sex education course may never initiate the behaviors required to do so. Also, poor verbal memory is common in schizophrenia (Goldman, Axelrod & Taylor, 1996) and therefore some patients simply may forget what they had intended to do. The solution to this particular problem would involve patients' primary nurses providing repeated reminders or prompts. Formal referrals by ward physicians would also increase the number educated but to date no patient has been referred (see the discussion about staff preparation above).

Additionally, patients may have been discouraged from attending the course or using the privacy suite by staff who were biased against the policy. Anecdotal reports suggest that this could have been a factor. For example, a rumor circulated among patients and staff that it "required a Ph.D. to pass the sex education course." This rumor was so prevalent that it was heard by one of the authors while attending a local conference from a professional not affiliated with Riverview! In fact there is no test and the course is tailored to suit each patient (the sex education course is discussed later). The solution to this problem is to better prepare staff for the implementation of the policy, as described above.

A third possible reason is related to the second. Although the sex education course was to be offered by several nurses on each ward, which in turn would give patients easy access to the course, this never materialized. Since the policy was implemented, several staff have provided sex education to patients but there has rarely been more than one educator available at any given time. Obviously a single educator can see a limited number of patients. Again, better staff preparation likely would generate interest by ward staff in teaching the course.

A number of patients who received education said they would be embarrassed to be seen entering the cottage containing the private suites. This is perplexing since patients had considerable input in selecting the cottage as the site for the suites and since some patients apparently are not embarrassed about engaging in sexual activity in more public places within the hospital. Again, we suspect that disapproval by some staff may be contributing to patient discomfort.

Table 5.1 is a summary of strategies that may be of help in the successful involvement of clinical staff, parents and patients in policy implementation.

Timing of Policy Implementation

At the time the policy was being formulated and implemented, Riverview was in the process of downsizing, was beginning to implement a psychosocial rehabilitation approach to the care and treatment

Table 5.1. Strategies for Involving the Key Groups in the Implementation of a Sexuality Policy.

Group	Approach	Strategy
Medical Staff	Decrease fear of litigation by emphasizing that the duty to protect patients is best achieved with a written policy that provides safeguards but does not prohibit sex.	Gain endorsement of the policy from the Medical Director. Provide sufficient question and answer sessions with a lawyer.
Nursing Staff	Emphasize that psychiatric nursing includes addressing patient sexuality. Emphasize the need for "safe sex" education to ensure that the policy is not viewed only as a vehicle for permitting sex.	Gain endorsement of the policy from the Nursing Administration. Provide at least 6 hours of education on the policy and its implementation. Encourage nursing staff to be responsible for arranging patient education.
Family Members	Emphasize the role of the policy in preventing HIV and unwanted pregnancies.	Discuss the policy and its implementation at family-support group meetings.
Patients	Emphasize that the policy recognizes patient needs for respect, dignity, and confidentiality. Facilitate access to education. Ensure that policy requirements are simple and manageable.	Provide sex education in a manner that reflects each patient's unique learning style. (e.g., content of curriculum, individual or group format, duration and location of sessions, degree of repetition, use of role playing, etc.)

of patients, and was holding meetings to evaluate the possible advantages of converting from department management to program management. Many nursing staff at the ward level felt uncertain about their future and unclear about their roles and responsibilities. In this climate of change and uncertainty, it was difficult to encourage or convince nursing staff that they should accept and embrace yet another significant change by implementing the sexuality policy, especially when this required that they become involved in an area of patient life that some preferred to ignore.

Change of any sort is frequently anxiety inducing and multiple institutional changes of any sort are likely to generate resistance. Ideally the types of institutional changes described above would occur one at a time, with time in-between to allow staff to adapt. It is probably unrealistic to expect this. However, fewer concurrent institutional changes and better staff preparation would likely help reduce resistance to any controversial new policy.

Sex Education Course

The task force was responsible for deciding the nature and extent of the sex education course offered to patients. As mentioned this course is a prerequisite to patient use of the private suites. There are indications in the literature that many patients with serious mental illness tend to score poorly on questionnaires that assess knowledge of HIV and risk behaviors (Goisman, Kent, Montgomery, Chevers & Goldfinger, 1992; Graham & Cates, 1992; Kalichman et al., 1994; Kelly et al., 1992) and there is some evidence that sex education classes increase knowledge scores in such patients (Berman & Rozensky, 1984; Goisman et al., 1992; Meyer et al., 1992). Consequently, it was not difficult to convince task force members to include the requirement for a sex education course in the policy. However there were differences in opinion as to what the curriculum should contain. For example, while a representative of the PES believed that the curriculum should include a heavy emphasis on safe sex practices, members of the Riverview Family Group felt strongly that the curriculum should include information about the genetic transmission of mental illness within the context of a discussion of contraception. Other members of the task force believed that patients should be taught reproductive anatomy and social skills. Ultimately the representative from the hospital's Mental Health Education Services prepared a curriculum that satisfied task force members and was similar to curricula described in the literature (Berman & Rozensky, 1984; Davidhizar et al., 1991; Goisman et al., 1991; Jacobs & Bobek, 1991; Lukoff et al., 1986; Meyer et al., 1992; Sladyk, 1990; Steiner, Lussier, Maust, DiPalma & Allende, 1994; Walker & Fraiser, 1994). The original course consisted of eight 30- to 60-minute sessions, taught to groups of six to eight patients. The original instructors were the representative from Riverview's Mental Health Education Services and the nurse clinician in the SRP.

A number of problems arose with the sex education course. Our difficulty persuading patients to attend the course has already been discussed, as has our failure to convince several nurses on each ward teach the course. The representative from Mental Health Education Services and the nurse clinician from SRP had been selected as educators on an interim basis until ward nurses were prepared to take over this duty, which never occurred. These two staff were required to return to their regular duties and then the Cottage Supervisor took on the role of educator. For most of the period since the policy's inception, this person alone has been responsible for all sex education. Problems associated with having a single educator were discussed earlier in the chapter.

Although group sex education formats have been described in the literature, many of the patients who volunteered to attend our course were not comfortable in a group. As would be expected, some also had difficulty concentrating and staying in the group for 30 to 60 minutes. Initially the course was provided in a special classroom in the cottage, with the plans to relocate it on the wards when ward nurses took over teaching. As discussed earlier, some patients expressed embarrassment about being seen entering the cottage.

For these reasons the original format of the sex education course was abandoned shortly after it was initiated. At present there is no specific format; patients are educated individually or in couples for sessions that last only as long as the patients' attention span, and education occurs in the cottage kitchen over coffee and cigarettes or on the patients' wards if that is their preference. It is probably true to say that no two patients receive the curriculum in an identical format. Rather, the course format is tailored to suit the needs of each patient and may change session by session. Duration, location and number of sessions are provided as needed by the patients. This greater flexibility appears to work well.

Although our curriculum was similar to those described in the literature, it proved to be too long and complicated for many of the patients. We now have two curricula, one basic and the other extended. The basic curriculum covers only information required to pass the competency test (see Welch & Clements, 1996). It does not include details such as reproductive anatomy or the menstrual cycle, for as Wasow (1980, p.15) has indicated, "plumbing lectures" tend to be beyond the ability and interest of many patients. The extended curriculum includes additional information on sex and relationships that a higher functioning patient may want to learn. Most of our patients are able to complete the basic curriculum, given our flexible delivery format.

Another problem with the course relates to an unintended association that formed in the minds of some patients and staff between the sex education course and the private suites. Although the course is a prerequisite to accessing the suites, the policy emphasizes that sex education should be available to all patients, even if they do not wish to use the private suites. Unfortunately the bias against the provision of private suites held by some staff (and probably some patients) appeared to become attached to the sex education course. Some staff and patients viewed the course only as a vehicle for using the suites rather than as a valuable experience in its own right. It is likely that this reduced the interest in the course for some patients. To solve this problem we are attempting to dissociate the sex education course from the private suites. We are attempting to teach patients and staff that volunteering for the course is not synonymous with using the private suites.

Additionally, although the value of sex education and HIV risk reduction courses for the mentally ill has been widely accepted (e.g., Bhui & Puffett, 1994; Cournos *et al.*, 1994; Woolf & Jackson, 1996), there is relatively little evidence that increases in knowledge, as measured by questionnaires, translate into behavior change. For example, Woolf & Jackson (1996) found that "those who showed good knowledge of safer sex practices functioned poorly at the practical skills of condom use..." (p. 302). McDermott, Sautter, Winstead and Quirk (1994) report, "No indications of a relationship between knowledge about AIDS and behavior change were found among the depressed or schizophrenic subjects" (p. 584). Meyer *et al.* (1992) found that, while knowledge scores on a questionnaire increased after participation in a psychoeducational program, there was no evidence of a concomitant increase in condom use. Brady and Carmen (1990) found that, "Most patients are able to comprehend the basic principles of risk reduction, but behavioral change is a slow and complex process" (p. 91). While we have found no guaranteed solution to this problem, there are therapeutic techniques that might increase the probability of behavior change. Since it is widely recognized that mentally handicapped persons of all kinds learn better by doing than by talking, the incorporation of role-playing (e.g., behavior rehearsal) into sex education groups may facilitate the occurrence of relevant behaviors such as assertively insisting that a partner use a condom, assertively saying no to combining drugs and sex, and using a condom properly (e.g., Goisman *et al.*, 1991; Meyer *et al.*, 1992). We incorporate behavior rehearsal into our curriculum whenever possible.

Encouraging Safe Sex Practices

Although instruction about condom use and provision of condoms to the chronically mental ill has met with opposition in some hospitals (e.g., Davidhizar *et al.*, 1991) and does not guarantee actual condom use (e.g., Meyer *et al.*, 1992), most sex education curricula for the mentally ill involve both provision of condoms and instruction in proper use (Walker & Fraiser, 1994; Goisman *et al.*, 1991). The Riverview Policy on Patient Sexuality states, "Condoms are freely available in all patient areas. Designated staff ensure that an adequate supply of condoms is available at all times." (p. 2). Because the PES representatives on the task force strongly objected, due to loss of privacy, to patients having to ask nurses for condoms, bowls of condoms were placed in male and female patient washrooms throughout the SRP and the recreation centre. Problems arose almost immediately. Condoms disappeared in remarkable numbers; at one time it was documented that between 200 and 300 condoms a day were vanishing from the recreation center. Condom dispensers were installed in each washroom with the hope that this would encourage patients to be more thoughtful about this behavior. However, condoms continued to vanish. Consideration was given to altering the condom machines so that they would require a minimal sum (such as a nickel) or a token. However, a PES representative objected that these measures would place an unnecessary obstacle in the way of patients and might discourage condom use. The disappearance of condoms was finally determined to be a cultural anomaly and hospital administration agreed to continue supplying an inordinate number. Members of the task force predicted that, as the novelty of an inexhaustible supply of condoms wore off, patients would lose interest in removing them from the washrooms. Fortunately, this proved to be the case.

As might be expected, the rapid disappearance of condoms resulted in condom dispensers often being empty. This fact was reported to the task force by a representative of the PES who regularly visited the patients washrooms on the wards and recreation center. A debate ensued about who should fill the condom dispensers. A PES representative proposed that the dispensers be filled on each shift by a member of the nursing staff and that a record be kept to ensure that this task was carried out. Nursing protested that this task was too time consuming and that it indicated a lack of trust in ward nurses. After lengthy discussion, this issue was resolved by assigning the task of filling the condom dispensers to the housekeeping staff. If dispensers ran out, patients were to report this to nursing staff.

Other problems emerged in regard to patients' access to condoms. Shortly after the condom dispensers were installed, it was discovered that someone had pricked holes in condoms, which were then left in the trays of the dispensers in the recreation center. Signs were posted warning patients to use only condoms that they dispensed themselves. Condoms already dispensed and left in the dispenser tray were to be examined by staff for signs of tampering and then disposed of. Not long after the warning signs went up, reports of tampering ceased.

Finally, a PES representative reported that the hospital had purchased condoms in packages that were difficult for patients to open or could not be opened without risk of damage. A different brand had to be ordered. Patients had been aware of the difficulty in opening the original brand for some time. This indicates the importance of consulting patients on all aspects of policy creation and implementation.

Davidhizar *et al.* (1991) reported that they dispensed condoms in plastic bins on the medicine cart and that their patients apparently did not mind this method of presentation even though it lacked anonymity. However, other researchers have reported problems with condoms similar to those experienced at Riverview. Woolf and Jackson (1996) found that patients never asked for condoms when they had to approach a nurse for them but did take condoms from a sex education group. Walker and Fraiser (1994) found that when condoms were placed in washrooms, patients frequently filled them with water and threw them around, resulting in complaints from visitors! These problems notwithstanding, condoms are a very important aspect of HIV risk reduction, and any hospital policy on patient sexuality must ensure that they are made available to patients in a manner that is acceptable to the patients at that hospital. It should be anticipated that various and unique problems will arise with the introduction of condoms to the wards. Our experience was that most problems were related to the novelty of having easy access to condoms and resolved as the novelty wore off.

Sexual Abuse Counseling

The Riverview Policy on Sexuality states, "Counseling for victims of sexual abuse is offered by qualified therapists on a referral basis." (p. 2). The prevalence of childhood sexual abuse in the seriously mentally ill, as well as its relation to mental disorders and HIV infection, is reviewed elsewhere in this volume. Consistent with the requirements of the policy, a contractor with expertise in the area of sexual abuse was hired to perform a needs assessment and to form a trauma services group. The trauma services group was to be composed of a clinical psychologist with expertise in sexual abuse assessment and treatment who consulted on a part-time basis, two half-time social workers, two half-time nurses, and one half-time occupational therapist. The psychologist was hired, two social workers were assigned to the project and training of the social workers by the psychologist was completed. Twenty Riverview patients received some form of needs assessment and/or sexual abuse counseling.

The sexual abuse counseling service proved to be controversial and, like other aspects of the policy, met with some resistance. When the hospital budget necessitated some service cuts, the funds for the trauma services contract was terminated. Fortunately, the problem of sexual abuse and the need for services for sexual abuse survivors has achieved a high profile in B.C. as elsewhere. Consequently, when active advocacy brought the loss of the service to the attention of senior provincial politicians, the hospital administration was quickly given reason to believe that funding for the service would be forthcoming in the near future.

Location and Supervision of the Private Suites

The task force was responsible for determining the location of the private suites. A cottage located near enough to the SRP building to be accessible but far enough away to offer some privacy was selected because it was acceptable to the PES, clinical staff, and administration. It is essential to remember that privacy for patients is an important consideration when selecting the location of private suites. While this may seem obvious, this simple dignity often is overlooked in hospital settings, especially when there is some cost attached to it, whether measured in dollars or inconvenience to staff.

Next the task force deliberated about the supervision of the private suites. In order to increase confidentiality and dignity, a PES representative suggested that the task of supervising the cottage be contracted out to an agency not otherwise involved in patient care. The reason was that this would reduce the likelihood of ward nurses knowing about, and possibly talking about, patients' sex lives, which was a concern to the PES. However, legal consultants advised the task force that Riverview Hospital would remain legally liable for activities occurring on hospital grounds and consequently recommended that the cottage supervisor be a hospital staff member. The PES reluctantly accepted this argument.

Granting Access to the Private Suites

The policy specifies that patients who complete the sex education course are eligible to apply for access to the private suites, and that access is to be granted by the treatment team unless there is a known medical or psychiatric contraindication. A form was created to document that these condition had been met and that access had been granted. The task force assumed that, consistent with hospital policy for documenting patients' ground privileges and visit leaves, it would be the patient's psychiatrist or ward physician who would sign the form. However, hospital physicians objected, stating that they needed to consult with the Canadian Medical Protective Association to determine issues of legal liability. Because most physicians were private contractors and were not employees of the hospital, some were concerned that the policy would not protect them from liability. Eventually the medical representative on the task force reported that many physicians would not sign a form authorizing access to the private suites but that they would be willing to write an order denying a patient access when this was warranted.

Although the Riverview physicians appeared to be generally supportive of the sex education course, the reluctance of some to authorize access to the private suites could only have served to increase anxiety and resistance among other staff. The physicians' expressed concern about legal liability probably increased the "litigaphobia" that already surrounded the patient sexuality policy.

When considering the validity of our physicians' fear of litigation it should be recalled again that physicians and other mental health professionals tend to significantly overestimate the risk of being sued (Brodsky, 1988; Lawthers *et al.*, 1992). Moreover, it may be argued that using a hospital-approved policy to assist in making a decision about a patient's expression of sexuality, as opposed to relying upon personal values and judgment, would help to protect any professional, whether an employee or contractor. This argument aside, a decision was made that allowed any willing member of a patient's treatment team to sign the form, which indicated that the team had approved a patient's request to use the private suites. Task force representatives added the phrase "signature on behalf of the treatment team" to the authorization form because this diffusion of responsibility appeared to reduce the anxiety of clinical members.

Identification of the Partner

Partners of patients granted access to the private suites could be other patients, probably from a different ward and granted access to the private suites by a different treatment team, or they could be significant others who were not hospital patients. Discussions were held about the need for a treatment team to know the identity of the partner after a patient had been granted access to the private suites. Representatives from the PES were against this as they believed it to be an unnecessary infringement on their privacy. However, the task force's medical representative argued that because some patients were perceived to be vulnerable to abuse by or the bad judgement of some partners, physicians would want the option of "disallowing" any particular partner (e.g., a partner who had provided a patient with illicit drugs). This led to considerable debate because some task force members felt that this action would serve to make an already conservative policy even less appealing to patients. The problem was resolved by adding several conditions to the form used to approve patient access to the private suites. The ability to "disallow" a particular partner exists but staff must document the reason why. Staff also must discuss the issue with the patient and consider the likely impact on the patient of disallowing a partner. That is, if the patient agrees that sexual intimacy with the partner would be bad for him or her, the decision to disallow is essentially made jointly with the patient. On the other hand, if the patient says or implies that he or she will have sex with the partner elsewhere in the hospital or on the grounds, the partner is not disallowed on the basis that a patient with a clinically undesirable partner will be safer in the private suite, where some degree of supervision is present, than in stairwells or bushes. This process allows staff to weigh all likely outcomes and select a course of action that is most in keeping with the combined objectives of patient autonomy and acting in the patients' best interest.

Responsibilities for Implementing the Policy

The policy requires certain actions of clinical staff. For example, a sexual history is to be taken, counseling for a variety of sexual issues is to be provided, sexual education is to be provided, and so on. Possibly due to resistance and possibly due to current workload, various aspects of the policy have not been implemented in a consistent manner. This problem was brought to the attention of hospital administration and the outcome was a 1997 revision of the policy to make it more succinct and comprehensible to staff, along with the creation of a related document, "Clinical Practice Guideline: Management of Patient Sexual Practices." This guideline specifies precisely and succinctly the responsibilities of individuals most directly involved in implementing the policy for any particular patient: nurse, physician, social worker, treatment team, cottage supervisor, and patient. This document has been included in each relevant Policy and Procedures Manual for a few months only, and its effect has yet to be evaluated. Our expectation is that this precise designation of responsibilities will help ensure that all aspects of the policy are implemented.

SUGGESTIONS FOR MORE EFFECTIVE IMPLEMENTATION

Implementation of the Riverview Hospital Policy on Patient Sexuality has been difficult, but valuable lessons were learned and the hospital administration remains committed to solving the problems encountered. Indeed, such a policy must be developed and implemented in spite of the many factors in existence at most psychiatric hospitals that work against it if we are to achieve for our patients an acceptable standard of care and a reasonable quality of life.

A retrospective analysis of the problems we encountered with policy implementation suggests that three specific actions might increase the likelihood of the policy's being accepted and utilized by both patients and staff. These actions are: (1) better preparing staff for the policy; (2) reconceptualizing the duty to protect in order to fulfil that duty in a manner that facilitates patient ability to use the private suites; and (3) enhancing patient motivation to attend sex education groups and to use the private suites for sexual intimacy, as opposed to stairwells and bushes. Before discussing these suggestions further, we need to caution that at this time the ideas presented below are those of the authors only; endorsement of these views by Riverview Hospital administration, clinical staff, patients, families, and other stakeholder groups is not implied. This caution made, it is noteworthy that a recent meeting of some senior clinical administrators resulted in considerable support for the ideas that follow.

Better Preparation of Staff

As indicated earlier, we believe that the considerable staff bias and resistance encountered at Riverview probably could have been circumvented to a large degree by better staff preparation about the policy and its implementation. Literature reviewed above suggests that a single 90-minute seminar was insufficient to both educate staff about their roles in policy implementation and to address their concerns and anxieties about patient sexuality. Moreover, the original plan for a one-day seminar per ward may have been too intensive. At other hospitals, a series of education sessions appears to have had a more desirable effect. Most sessions described in the literature were 90 minutes although one was reported to be 2 1/2 hours. The number of sessions in a series ranged from four to eight. The total number of hours devoted to staff education ranged from 6 to 15.

Better staff preparation, with subsequent reduction in bias and resistance, not only should facilitate staff participation in policy implementation, but also could translate into greater patient participation in the sex education course and use of the private suites, with the latter presumably reducing the numbers of sexual liaisons occurring in unsafe locations. This desirable effect on patients would be expected because a more enthusiastic clinical staff would likely be more attentive to their responsibilities under the policy, more attentive to patient sexual needs, more likely to suggest or refer patients for sex education, more likely to provide patients with sex education and less anxious about encouraging sexually active patients to use the private suites.

An increased number of staff education sessions obviously would require a capital expense. However, from a purely financial perspective, if successful implementation of the policy has the effect of reducing the prevalence of HIV infection in the hospital, the savings in health dollars over the lifetime of those patients would more than offset the cost of staff preparation. Of course from a clinical care as well as an ethical perspective, prevention of one case of HIV infection or one unwanted pregnancy would justify the expense.

Reconceptualizing the Duty to Protect

The Riverview Policy on Patient Sexuality contains a number of provisions designed to protect patients from harm while using the private suites. Before using the suites, all patients must participate in the sex education course, patients with a medical contraindication such as HIV seropositivity are not allowed to use the suites, and patients with a psychiatric contraindication (inability to consent or engage in safe sex) as determined by a formal test of capability, are not allowed to use the suites. These provisions of the policy no doubt served to reduce litigation anxiety in administration, clinical staff, and family members, but, given our experience with the policy to date, we have begun to doubt that any policy provision that prevents patients from accessing the private suites necessarily serves to protect them from harm. Rather, these provisions might have the opposite effect; they might increase the probability of some patients engaging in risky sexual behavior. To understand our argument, it is necessary to accept as true two premises.

First, it is safer for patients to engage in sexual activity in private suites such as those at Riverview than in stairwells, bushes, or similar places in the hospital. There are several reasons to believe this. The private suites contain condoms at the bedside and provide clear reminders to use them in the form of the visible presence of the condoms themselves, posters on safe sex, and reminders from the Cottage Supervisor. Also, even though the patients have been granted access to the suites by the treatment team, the Cottage Supervisor sees the patients at the time they arrive to use the suites and can take whatever action is reasonable if either patient appears to be intoxicated, grossly psychotic, or coerced to use the suite. Finally, the suites contain a "panic button" and the Cottage Supervisor is downstairs, should any problem occur in the suite. Of course stairwells, bushes, and similar places do not contain any of the above. Our contention then, is that sex in a private suite always is safer for patients than sex elsewhere on hospital grounds.

Second, denying a sexually active patient access to a private suite for any reason increases the likelihood that the patient will engage in sex elsewhere. There is no reason to believe that denying access to a private suite will prevent a sexually active patient from finding another location. To the contrary, data reviewed earlier in this chapter indicate that many patients are sexually active while in hospital in the absence of private suites. Although it is equally true that allowing patients to have sex in private suites does not prevent them from having sex elsewhere as well, it is reasonable to assume that patients would prefer the comfort of the suites, and, if they were always allowed access to the suites, it is reasonable to assume that some degree of sexual satiation would occur and reduce the likelihood of sexual activity occurring elsewhere.

If these two premises are true, then it may be necessary to reconceptualize how we can best protect patients from harm. We suggest the following:

1. The policy on patient sexuality must continue to emphasize the importance of sex education (including HIV risk reduction techniques) with flexible formats and curricula that best meet the needs of each patient. Nurses should make an effort to provide sex education to a new patient as soon as the patient is sufficiently stabilized, and they should document this. However, it should not be mandatory for a patient to complete a formal course before access to a private suite is allowed. The time required to complete a course is time the patient is at risk. Moreover, not all sexually active patients will agree to attend a course, and those who refuse will be placed at increased risk if denied access to a suite.

2. The policy must continue to emphasize the importance of assessing patients' sexual needs, including areas such as HIV risk behavior, HIV testing, birth control, sexual abuse, and sexual dysfunction. Appropriate counseling should be available as needed. The assessment should be performed by any member of the treatment team the patient is comfortable with and who in turn is comfortable discussing sexual issues. The assessment should be performed in an atmosphere of calm and openness to facilitate the patient's ability to talk about sexual issues. Guidelines for talking to patients about sexual matters are available (Bor & Watts, 1993) and will not be discussed further here. Our primary point is that clinical staff should make a consistent effort to establish trust and increase the probability of the patient's making a decision to do what is in his or her best interest with regard to obtaining education, counseling and reducing HIV risk behavior. Openness, a nonjudgmental attitude, and other elements of a good therapeutic relationship will not have undesirable effects such as increasing the likelihood of a patient engaging in unprotected sex in the bushes but might result in a patient abstaining from sex until adequately educated.

3. A formal test of capability to consent and behave responsibly should be replaced by an informal but documented assessment by the Cottage Supervisor, which occurs at the time a patient arrives at the suite. The presumption of capability should apply unless clinical observation (e.g., signs of intoxication, grossly disorganized behavior, fearful behavior) or a brief verbal assessment (e.g., "Mary, you look confused. Do you know why you are here?") suggest that a patient may be incapable of consenting or behaving responsibly at that time when the patient arrives to use the suite (recall that the Cottage Supervisor is a nurse who has the clinical skills to assess for possible indicators of incapability).

4. Since any patient might want to use the private suites, the Cottage Supervisor should be made a member of each patient's treatment team. This would permit the Cottage Supervisor to be informed if a particular patient is known to be HIV positive because this information is documented in the patient's medical chart and is available to

members of the treatment team. Patients who are HIV positive should
not be denied access to the suites; they are more likely to infect other
patients if they have sex in stairwells and bushes. However, it is
likely that the Cottage Supervisor would be legally obligated to require these patients to disclose their HIV status to their partners
before accessing the suite (see legal considerations, below).
5. Points 1–4 above would negate the need for a formal application
   form for access to the private suites.

Enhancing Patient Motivation

Some patients with mental illness such as schizophrenia will remain
apathetic, have difficulty inhibiting a sexual impulse, or find it difficult to initiate the required behaviors when the time to attend a sex
education course, walk to the private suite, or put on a condom arises.
Can anything be done to increase the probability of these behaviors?
Outside the realm of sex, there are many examples of the success of
behavioral techniques (e.g., positive reinforcement, token economies)
in motivating patients with schizophrenia to engage in desirable behaviors (Bellack & Mueser, 1993; Paul & Lentz, 1977). A review of the
behavioral literature is beyond the scope of this chapter but suffice it to
say that behavioral techniques such as the provision of prompts by
nurses and positive reinforcement by course instructors might serve to
increase attendance and participation in sex education sessions. Use
of private suites could be directly reinforced with patients who are
known or suspected of being sexually active elsewhere in the hospital
or grounds. While this does not preclude having sex elsewhere, increased use of a private suite is likely to be associated with a degree of
satiation of the sex drive and this in turn might reduce sexual activity
elsewhere. Condom use could be directly reinforced. In the private suites
at Riverview, special receptacles are available for disposing of used
condoms. With patient consent, these receptacles would allow for the
monitoring of condom use before and after the initiation of a positive
reinforcement intervention.

Although these ideas may seem provocative, the challenge to mental health professionals of reducing HIV risk behaviors and the spread
of HIV in the seriously mentally ill will undoubtedly require novel and
perhaps controversial approaches. Observing used condoms may not
be an appealing prospect but nurses certainly carry out other unap-
pealing procedures when caring for special populations such as the
elderly with dementia or persons with severe mental handicaps.

LEGAL CONSIDERATIONS

Noffsinger in this volume has discussed legal considerations related
to sex and mental illness within an American context. Because we

have described a policy developed in a Canadian psychiatric hospital, a brief discussion of relevant Canadian law is prudent to avoid possible confusion to readers about the two legal systems. Of course, one country's laws can be of theoretical interest and persuasive value at the other side of the border, as we hope proves to be the case for American readers. While detailed legal arguments regarding B.C. and Canadian laws are not appropriate here, Canadian readers should still find this section to be of practical value.

Legal Support for the Riverview Policy on Patient Sexuality

Two main questions must be considered from a legal perspective:

1. Do psychiatric inpatients have a legal right to sexual intimacy in a private and dignified setting, as we have contended?
2. Does the hospital have a legal duty to protect patients from harm that may arise from sexual interactions?

We will briefly address each of these questions below.

In the Canadian context there is no need to argue that "sexual interaction per se [is] a specifically protected right" (Perlin, 1993, p. 530). The common law's position is that a person is free to do anything that is not positively prohibited (Hogg, 1992). It goes without saying that, with the exception of various Criminal Code provisions dealing with consent, there is no such prohibition of sexual interaction anywhere. If it were necessary to argue that the right to exercise sexual intimacy is derived from statute, this would almost certainly be based on the *Canadian Charter of Rights and Freedoms* (1982), which is part of the Canadian Constitution. Until very recently, it was almost impossible to argue that the Charter applies to hospitals since they are not part of or directly controlled by government (Welch & Clements, 1996). However, in *Eldridge* v *British Columbia* (1997) the Supreme Court of Canada has now concluded that when hospitals provide services to patients that are mandated under legislation, they are acting as the vehicle chosen by government to achieve its objectives so that the Charter does apply in this respect. Since it is now clear that hospital patients and, a *fortiori*, involuntary psychiatric patients have charter-protected rights, would these rights include that of sexual interaction?

What follows is an extremely cursory reference to relevant key sections of the Charter, a detailed consideration of which is well beyond the scope of this chapter. Section 7 grants "Everyone...the right to life, liberty and security of the person and the right not to be deprived thereof except in accordance with the principles of fundamental justice." Both the liberty and the security of the person's rights are involved with respect to involuntary psychiatric patients; the latter because of the removal of aspects of control over one's body (see Hogg, 1992, p. 44-10).

It is noteworthy that the word "control" is part of the involuntary commital criteria in section 22 of the B.C. *Mental Health Act*. In addition, section 15 entitles individuals to "the right to the equal protection and equal benefit of the law without discrimination based on ...mental...disability." The Supreme Court of Canada considered the effect of section 15 with respect to physical disability in *Eldridge*, above, in connection with the right of persons with hearing impairments to interpreters in hospitals. We submit that similar reasoning can be applied to persons with a mental disability.

A note of caution is warranted, however, because of the so-called judicial override clause in section 1 of the Charter. This allows a judge to determine that, despite the means used being a violation of a Charter-protected right, a government objective may be so important that it can be "demonstrably justified". However, this argument was unsuccessful in *Eldridge*.

We conclude, therefore, that a good argument can be made that hospitals owe patients a duty to enable them to exercise their right of sexual intimacy in a private and dignified setting. For a detailed discussion of various relevant Charter decisions of the Supreme Court of Canada, we refer to Hogg (1992).

Turning now to a hospital's duty to protect, the Policy on Patient Sexuality requires patients to be capable of consenting to sex and behaving responsibly before being granted access to a private suite. Under common law, capability must be presumed unless indicators of possible incapability are present. This presumption is also recognized under B.C.'s *Adult Guardianship Act*. Nevertheless, there can be no doubt that part of the standard of care that a hospital owes to its patients is the duty to protect patients from harming themselves or others. This is clear from both the common law and Section 3 of the *Occupiers Liability Act* .

Any liability arising out of a successful action on account of breach of the duty to protect could be direct (for physicians with admitting privileges and other independent contractors), vicarious (for the hospital on behalf of its employees), and what has traditionally been termed direct liability on the part of the institution itself but is now most frequently referred to in the literature as corporate liability. Corporate liability could arise out of action of the governing board itself, or more likely out of a failure to have a proper policy, system, or organization in place. It is our contention, also expressed elsewhere in this chapter that the existence of the kind of policy as discussed here is more likely to reduce the potential for direct, vicarious, and corporate liability than to increase it. Since the institution is aware, as it must be unless it is wilfully blind, that some of its patients have sex with each other or with visitors, its duty to protect patients and visitors is more easily discharged by making efforts to educate patients, considering their capability to use a private suite and providing a supervised, private place to conduct sexual activities where educational material and condoms are available. A formal policy should protect employees (Welch & Clements, 1996) and may even assist independent contractors provide a sound basis for their decisions regarding patient sexuality.

Legal Support for Reconceptualized Duty to Protect

In an earlier section of this paper we indicated that our experience with the Riverview Policy on Patient Sexuality had caused us to reconceptualize the duty to protect. Is our suggested reconceptualization legally defensible? We believe so for the reasons presented below.

Although it is obviously preferable from a legal perspective to make it mandatory to attend sex education classes and to pass a capability test, if this causes patients to shun the private suites and to continue to use stairwells and the hospital grounds, this makes it impossible for the hospital to discharge its duty of care which, in B.C., is coupled with the duty to supervise and control which arises out of the committal criteria in the *Mental Health Act*. Surely it cannot be seriously argued that the duty to protect should be discharged by policing the grounds and stairwells and prohibiting sexual activity within the hospital environment. This would be contrary to law as well as, we submit, basic ethical principles and common sense.

The presence of a Cottage Supervisor in the building would allow informal assessment for capacity to give consent to sexual activity and to engage in safer sexual practices. Moreover, it is arguable that to carry out his or her duties in a responsible manner, the Cottage Supervisor should be a member of the treatment team of all patients. Nothing in the provincial *Freedom of Information and Protection of Privacy Act* prevents the Cottage Supervisor from thus having access to patients' records since this would follow from a "need to know" to carry out his or her function in this respect. This would permit the Cottage Supervisor to have knowledge of, and be able to warn patients about, potential harm arising from factors such as the HIV positive status of particular partners. As to whether B.C. law imposes a duty to warn an individual that the person with whom they propose to share a private suite is HIV positive, this is not free from doubt. There is clearly a general duty to warn or otherwise protect individuals in circumstances where harm to those individuals is reasonably foreseeable (Robertson, 1994). However, it seems that a good case can be made that in the type of situation under discussion the likelihood of harm is greater if confidentiality is breached if this induces the HIV positive partner to avoid use of the private suites. It strains common sense to believe that patients will refrain from sex if they choose not to use a private suite because this becomes too unattractive. There can be little doubt that in general patients will be safer using a suite because of the presence of the supervisor in the building, the consequent opportunity for informal observation and inquiry regarding possible incapability, the possibility for intervention in case of emergency and the availability of condoms. However, in the end it remains to be said that because of the preoccupation of tort law with compensation for the individual who has suffered foreseeable harm (*Wenden* v. *Trikha*, 1993), it is more likely than not that a court would find liability on the part of a hospital that was aware of a patient's HIV positivity when that patient chose to use a private suite and the hospital did not warn the partner of this.

REFERENCES

Adult Guardianship Act, R.S.B.C. 1996, c.6 (not yet in force).

Akhtar, S., Crocker, E., Dickey, N., Helfrish, J. & Rheuban, W. (1977). Overt sexual behavior among psychiatric inpatients. *Diseases of the Nervous System* 38:359–361.

Alexander, M. (1988). Clinical determination of mental competence. *Archives of Neurology* 45:23–26.

Bell, C., Wringer, P., Davidhizar, R. & Samuels, M. (1993). Self-reported sexual behaviors of schizophrenic clients and noninstitutionalized adults. *Perspectives in Psychiatric Care* 29:30–36.

Bellack, A. & Mueser, K. (1993). Psychosocial treatment for schizophrenia. *Schizophrenia Bulletin* 19:317–336.

Berman, C. & Rozensky, R. (1984). Sex education for the chronic psychiatric patient: The effects of a sexual-issues group on knowledge and attitudes. *Psychosocial Rehabilitation Journal* 8:29–33.

Bhui, K. & Puffett, A. (1994). Sexual problems in the psychiatric and mentally handicapped populations. *British Journal of Hospital Medicine* 51:459–464.

Bor, R. & Watts, M. (1993). Talking to patients about sexual matters. *British Journal of Nursing* 2:657–661.

Brady, S. & Carmen, E. (1990). AIDS risk in the chronically mentally ill: Clinical strategies for prevention. *New Directions in Mental Health Services* 48: 83–95.

Brodsky, S. (1988). Fear of litigation in mental health professionals. *Criminal Justice and Behavior* 15:492–500.

Canadian Charter of Rights and Freedoms. Constitution Act; 1982.

Canadian Council on Health Facilities Accreditation (1994). *Accreditation Survey Report*. Ottawa: Author.

Civic, D., Walsh, G. & McBride, D. (1990). Staff perspectives on sexual behavior of patients in a state psychiatric hospital. *Hospital and Community Psychiatry* 35:765–768.

Cohen, D. & Tanenbaum, R. (1985). Sexuality education for staff in long-term psychiatric hospitals. *Hospital and Community Psychiatry* 36:187–189.

Commons, M., Bohn, J., Godon, L., Hauser, M. & Gutheil, T. (1992). Professional's attitudes towards sex between institutionalized patients. *American Journal of Psychotherapy* 46:571–580.

Cournos, F., Empfield, M., Horwath, E. & Kramer, M. (1986). The management of HIV infection in state psychiatric hospitals. *Hospital and Community Psychiatry* 40:153–157.

Cournos, F., Empfield, M., Horwath, E., McKinnon, K., Meyer, I., Schrage, H., Currie, C. & Agosin, B. (1991). HIV seroprevalence among patients admitted to two psychiatric hospitals. *American Journal of Psychiatry* 148: 1225–1230.

Cournos, F., Guido, J., Coomaraswamy, S., Meyer-Bahlburg, H., Sugden, R.& Horwath, E. (1994). Sexual activity and risk of HIV infection among patients with schizophrenia. *American Journal of Psychiatry* 151:228-232.
Davidhizar, R., Boonstra, C., Lutz, K. & Poston, P. (1991). Teaching safer sex in a long-term psychiatric setting. *Perspectives in Psychiatric Care* 27: 25-29.
Eldridge v. *B.C.* (1997), 151 D.L.R.(4th) 577(S.C.C.)
Firn, S. (1994) No sex please....*Nursing Times* 90:14.
Fleishchhacker, W., Meise, U., Gunther, V. & Kurz, M. (1994). Compliance with antipsychotic drug treatment: Influence of side effects. *Acta Psychiatrica Scandinavica* 89:11-15.
Freedman, M., Stuss, D. & Gordon, M. (1991). Assessment of competency: The role of neurobehavioral deficits. *Annals of Internal Medicine* 155:203-208.
Freedom of Information and Protection of Privacy Act, R.S.B.C. 1996, c.165.
Gitlin, M. (1994). Psychotropic medications and their effects on sexual function: Diagnosis, biology, and treatment approaches. *Journal of Clinical Psychiatry* 55:406-413.
Goisman, R., Kent, A., Montgomery, E., Cheevers, M. & Goldfinger, S. (1991). AIDS education for patients with chronic mental illness. *Community Mental Health Journal* 27:189-197.
Goldman, R., Axelrod, B. & Taylor, S. (1996). Neuropsychological aspects of schizophrenia. In I. Grant & K. Adams (Eds.), *Neuropsychological assessment of neuropsychiatric disorders* (2nd ed.) (pp.504-525) New York: Oxford University Press.
Goodman, L., Rosenberg, S., Mueser, K. & Drake, R. (1997). Physical and sexual assault history in women with serious mental illness: Prevalence, correlates, treatment, and future research directions. *Schizophrenia Bulletin* 23:685-696.
Gottesman, I. & Groome, C. (1997). HIV/AIDS risks as a consequence of schizophrenia. *Schizophrenia Bulletin* 23:675-684.
Graham, L. & Cates, J. (1992). How to reduce the risk of HIV infection for the seriously mentally ill. *Journal of Psychosocial Nursing* 30:9-13.
Hogg, P. (1992) *Constitutional law of Canada* (3rd ed.), Toronto, ON: Carswell; Thomson Canada Ltd.
Holbrook, T. (1989). Policing sexuality in a modern state hospital. *Hospital and Community Psychiatry* 40:75-79.
Jacobs, P., & Bobeck, S. (1991). Sexual needs of the schizophrenic client. *Perspectives in Psychiatric Care* 27:15-20.
Jacobson, M. & Herald, C. (1990). The relevance of childhood sexual abuse to adult psychiatric inpatient care. *Hospital and Community Psychiatry* 41:154-158.
Kalichman, S., Kelly, J., Johnson, J. & Bulto, M. (1994). Factors associated with risk for HIV infection among chronic mentally ill adults. *American Journal of Psychiatry* 151:221-227.
Keitner, G. & Grof, P. (1981). Sexual and emotional intimacy between psychiatric in-patients: Formulating a policy. *Hospital and Community Psychiatry* 32:188-193.
Kelly, J., Murphy, D., Bahr, R., Brasfield, T., Davis, D., Hauth, A., Morgan, M., Stevenson, L. & Eilers, M. (1992). AIDS/HIV risk behavior among the chronic mentally ill. *American Journal of Psychiatry* 149:886-889.
Lawthers, A., Localio, A., Laird, N., Lipsitz, S., Herbert, L. & Brennan, T. (1992). Physicians perceptions of the risk of being used. *Journal of Health Politics, Policy and Law* 17:463-482.
Leichtman, M. (1990). Attitudes of staff members toward a sex education program for hospitalized adolescents. *Bulletin of the Menninger Clinic* 54: 34-47.

Lukoff, D., Gioia-Hasick, D., Sullivan, G., Golden, J. & Nuerchterlein, K. (1986). Sex education and rehabilitation with schizophrenic male outpatients. *Schizophrenia Bulletin* 12:669–677.

McDermott, B., Sautter, F., Winstead, D. & Quirk, T. (1994). Diagnosis, health beliefs, and risk of HIV infection in psychiatric patients. *Hospital and Community Psychiatry* 45:580–585.

McSherry, B. & Somerville, A. (1996). *Sexual activity among institutionalized persons in need of special care.* Unpublished manuscript, McGill Centre for Medicine, Ethics and Law.

Mental Health Act, R.S.B.C. 1996, c.288.

Meyer, I., Cournos, F., Empfield, M., Agosin, B. & Floyd, P. (1992). HIV prevention among psychiatric inpatients: A pilot risk reduction study. *Psychiatric Quarterly* 63:187–197.

Meyer, I., McKinnon, K., Cournos, F., Empfield, M., Bavli, S., Engel, D. & Weinstock, A. (1993). HIV seroprevalence among long-stay patients in a state psychiatric hospital. *Hospital and Community Psychiatry* 44:282–284.

Nasrallah, H. (1992). The neuropsychiatry of schizophrenia. In S. Yudolsky & R. Hales (Eds.), *Textbook of neuropsychiatry* (2nd ed.)(pp.621–638). Washington, D.C.: American Psychiatric Press, Inc.

Occupiers Liability Act, R.S.B.C. 1996, c.337.

Ombudsman for the Province of British Columbia (1994). *Public report no. 33. Listening: A review of Riverview Hospital.* Victoria: Queen's Printer.

Paul, G. & Lentz., R. (1977). *Psychosocial treatment of chronic mental patients: Milieu versus social learning program.* Cambridge: Harvard University Press.

Perlin, M. (1993). Hospitalized patients and the right to sexual interaction: Beyond the last frontier? *New York University Review of Law and Social Change* 20:517–547.

Riverview Hospital Charter of Patient Rights (1994). Port Coquitlam, B.C.: Riverview Hospital.

Robertson, G. (1994). *Mental disability and the law in Canada,* (2nd ed) (pp.458–464). Scarborough, ON: Carswell; Thomson Canada Ltd.

Shaul, S. & Morrey, L. (1980). Sexuality education in a state mental hospital. *Hospital and Community Psychiatry* 31:175–179.

Sladyk, K. (1990). Teaching safe sex practices to psychiatric patients. *The American Journal of Occupational Therapy* 44:284–286.

Steiner, J., Lussier, R., Maust, G., DiPalma, L. & Allende, M. (1994). Psychoeducation about sexual issues in an acute treatment setting. *Hospital and Community Psychiatry* 45:380–381.

Trudel, G. & Desjardin, M. (1992). Staff reactions toward the sexual behaviors of people living in institutional settings. *Sexuality and Disability* 10:173–188.

Vandereycken, W. (1993). Shrinking sexuality: The half-known sex life of psychiatric patients. *Therapeutic Communities* 14:143–150.

Volavka, J., Convit, A., O'Donnell, J., Douyon, R., Evanelista, C. & Czobor, P. (1992). Assessment of risk behaviors for HIV infection among psychiatric inpatients. *Hospital and Community Psychiatry* 43:482–485.

Walker, S. & Fraiser, P. (1994). HIV and the long-term mentally ill. *Nursing Standard* 8:51–53.

Wasow, M. (1980). Sexuality and the institutionalized mentally ill. *Sexuality and Disability* 3:3–16.

Welch, S. & Clements, G. (1996). Development of a policy on sexuality for hospitalized chronic psychiatric patients. *Canadian Journal of Psychiatry* 41:273–279.

Wenden v. Trikha (1993). 14 C.C.L.T. (2d) 225 (Alberta Court of Appeal).

Withersty, D. (1976). Sexual attitudes of hospital personnel: A model for continuing education. *American Journal of Psychiatry* 133:573–575.

Wolfe, S. & Menninger, W. (1973). Fostering open communication about sexual concerns in a mental hospital. *Hospital and Community Psychiatry* 24:147–151.

Woolf, L. & Jackson, B. (1996). 'Coffee & Condoms': The implementation of a sexual health programme in acute psychiatry in an inner city area. *Journal of Advanced Nursing* 23:299–304.

6

Teaching Individuals with Serious Mental Illness About Friendship, Dating and Sexuality

ALEX KOPELOWICZ, ROBERT G. MANGANO and MITCH CAINE

INTRODUCTION

Individuals with serious and persistent mental illness present a disparate range of disabling symptoms, which interfere with cognitive and perceptual processes, affect, social functioning and behavior. Comprehensive biopsychosocial rehabilitation programs have been designed to overcome the multitude of deficits manifested by many of these individuals (Kopelowicz, Corrigan, Wallace & Liberman, 1996; Liberman, 1992). Each component of a biopsychosocial rehabilitative program is targeted toward one or more deficient areas of functioning in an effort to meet the individual's identified needs. For example, one such component, social skills training, is a structured application of behavioral learning principles aimed at helping individuals with serious mental illness build a repertoire of skills that improve their ability to function in the community. There is ample evidence that optimal biopsychosocial treatment and rehabilitation, when offered in a coordinated, comprehensive, and continuous fashion, can facilitate symptomatic and social recovery from schizophrenia and other disabling mental disorders (Kopelowicz & Liberman, 1994; Liberman, Wallace, Blackwell, Eckman, Vaccaro & Kuehnel, 1993).

The spectrum of services included within the domain of biopsychosocial rehabilitation has broadened with the increased recognition by practitioners that the goals of individuals with serious mental illness closely parallel the goals of individuals without psychiatric disorders. These aspirations include the desire to get an education, to work, to live independently, to have friends, to form intimate relationships, and to engage in sexual behavior (Uttaro & Mechanic, 1994). Of these functioning areas, the topic of sexuality has been given the least attention in this population (Kopelowicz, 1994). This neglect has historical roots, and may reflect a bias on the part of psychiatric practitioners, in that they may avoid exploration of sexual issues due to their own discomfort (Withersty, 1976; Coverdale & Aruffo, 1992), are concerned that the recognition of sexuality may trigger or implicitly condone inappropriate sexual behavior (Wasow, 1980), or assume that seriously mentally ill persons do not have active sex lives (McEvoy, Hatcher, Applebaum & Abernethy, 1983; Pinderhughes, Grace & Reyna, 1972). As recently as ten years ago, the sexual behavior of people with schizophrenia, especially men, was thought to be predominantly auto-erotic, with few sexual partners (Lukoff, Gioia-Hasick, Sullivan & Golden & Nuechterlein, 1986). However, more recent studies show that 60–70% of adults with serious mental illness report being sexually active in the past year (Laumann, Gagnon, Michael & Michaels, 1994), with approximately 30% reporting two or more partners (Buckley et al., Chapter 4, Carey, Carey, Weinhardt & Gordon, 1997).

Another reason that increased attention has been devoted to the sexuality of individuals with serious mental illness is their increased risk for human immunodeficiency virus (HIV) infection (McKinnon and Cournos, Chapter 7). The susceptibility for HIV among the seriously mentally ill has led the Centers for Disease Control to identify this group as high risk (Kalichman, Carey & Carey, 1996). Individuals with serious mental illness engage in a variety of high risk behaviors at higher rates than control groups, including not using a condom during sexual intercourse; sex with anonymous partners; trading sex for material gain; substance abuse in general and intravenous drug use specifically; and male homosexual activity (Carey et al., 1997). Moreover, individuals with serious mental illness may manifest hypersexuality during psychotic episodes (Akhtar & Thomson, 1980), and may lack the social skills necessary to decline sexual overtures, a finding particularly salient for its impact on women who are mentally ill (Friedman & Harrison, 1984).

Still another factor fueling the concern of practitioners for their patients' sexual behaviors is that most antipsychotic medications exert significant adverse influence on sexual drive and activity. Given that side effects are the most common reason for non-compliance with antipsychotic medication (Weiden, Aquila & Standard, 1996), sexual side effects such as ejaculatory difficulties, erectile dysfunction, decreased libido, orgasmic dysfunction, and priapism may play a pivotal role in the overall success of treatment (Millner *et al.*, Chapter 10). This is an area of neglect by most psychiatrists (Deegan, Chapter 2).

Sex-Related Interventions Targeted to the Seriously Mentally Ill

Clearly, sex education should be an integral part of a comprehensive rehabilitation program. Unfortunately, until recently this aspect of rehabilitation has been neglected. The current impetus for increasing patients' sexual knowledge is most certainly the alarmingly high rates of HIV found among the seriously mentally ill. Not surprisingly, the majority of sex education programs have been designed to increase patients' awareness of the risk of HIV and provide them with the knowledge and skills needed to decrease their chances of becoming infected (e.g., by teaching them how and why to use condoms). A few programs have had broader goals such as increasing patients' knowledge and comfort about sexuality, helping patients identify and clarify their values and attitudes about sexuality, helping patients acquire decision-making skills regarding sexual activity, and improving intimacy skills.

Many of the earliest published reports on sex-related interventions targeted to the seriously mentally ill did little more than describe the programs utilized and give anecdotal reports of their effectiveness (Friedman, 1976; Jones, 1983; Wasow, 1980). These pilot programs were useful in that they demonstrated that the seriously mentally ill were receptive to such topics and amenable to treatment focused on sexual issues. Additionally, this first generation of reports provided a framework of success upon which later, more systematic research could build. For example, Lukoff and colleagues created a sex education program within a comprehensive rehabilitation program for individuals with serious mental illness (Lukoff *et al.*, 1986). Patients attended eight biweekly one-hour sessions, which provided general sex education, including information on birth control and the prevention of sexually transmitted diseases, discussions intended to assist the participants in defining their own feelings toward sexual issues, ways to overcome medication-induced sexual dysfunction, and rudimentary training in intimacy skills. As part of this skills training, role-playing, modeling, and group exercises were used to teach decision-making skills related to finding partners and communication skills to maintain relationships and initiate appropriate discussions of physical intimacy.

Lukoff and colleagues utilized no control group and no outcome data was obtained, but participants reported enjoying the program, particularly the opportunity to discuss sexual issues. The authors noted that none of the participants experienced a relapse or exacerbation of symptoms, a fear that had previously been voiced by mental health professionals as a justification for not providing programs of a sexual nature in the rehabilitation process. In their discussion, the authors recommended that enhanced training in intimacy skills might contribute to improvements in sexual functioning.

The skills needed for romantic and physically intimate relationships was the focus of a program conducted in a group format for two hours per week over a six-month period (Howden, Zipple & Tyrrell, 1994). The group leaders encouraged participants to role-play those skills related to successful dating, such as initiating and maintaining conversations, arranging for transportation and planning dates on a limited income, accepting rejection, and skills related to sexual intercourse. AIDS and sex education were not specifically planned for but were discussed as these topics arose naturally in the course of group discussions.

As in the previous report, no control group was utilized or outcome data collected, but the authors reported that the group was enormously popular and there were anecdotal comments attesting to the effectiveness of the program. It is of interest to point out that in light of the comprehensive skills training provided, the authors recommended that such formal skills training should comprise no more than 35% of group time, so that there could be ample time to focus on supportive group discussions.

With the recognition in the early 1990s of the threat of HIV infection among those with serious mental illness (Carey, Weinhardt & Carey, 1995), issues of sexuality increasingly found their way into comprehensive psychiatric rehabilitation programming, albeit from the standpoint of sex education and HIV prevention. Descriptions of these HIV prevention programs can be classified into three categories, each category differing as a function of the scientific rigor employed to ascertain program efficacy.

The first category consisted of a series of anecdotal reports describing the programs utilized, providing suggestions for future programs, and not evaluated with respect to outcome. One such HIV prevention program included an AIDS risk assessment at intake, which set the tone for a frank discussion of sexual issues, and incorporated the acquired information into the individual's treatment plan. The intervention was a one-hour long, drop-in psychoeducational group available to both sexes with a didactic format that was fluid and responded to the interests and needs of its participants. The material covered varied according to the knowledge level of those in attendance, and included rudimentary information on AIDS and ways to decrease the risk of HIV infection, instruction and practice in condom use, individualized risk assessment for sexually transmitted diseases, and discussions of the emotional consequences of knowing someone who died from AIDS-related complications. While no formal data was collected, anecdotal evidence from group members suggested that the participants were able to make changes in HIV risk behaviors. Moreover, the open discussion of sexual issues permeated into many of the participants' other therapeutic activities. For example, clinicians noted that participants were more forthcoming about problems with substance abuse and medication noncompliance after the intervention (Brady and Carmen, 1990).

Davidhizar and colleagues (1991) conducted a strictly educational program implemented in a long-term psychiatric setting. The participants watched videos and were provided information on sex education, including HIV infection, and safer sex practices. No training in behavioral or social skills was provided. True/false questionnaires were given following the educational videos, but the results of these measures were not reported.

Graham and Cates (1992) used an intervention focused on AIDS education with 39 patients at a local community mental health center. Three one-hour sessions were conducted over a two week period, each session beginning with a 30-minute videotape followed by a discussion. Because some participants reported an increase in symptoms during the program and others had a difficult time assimilating the information, this format was considered less effective for teaching HIV risk-reduction techniques.

The second category of HIV prevention programs employed more formal evaluations to measure efficacy. For example, Goisman and colleagues (1991) provided 50 outpatients with three one-hour sessions covering sex education; information about AIDS, such as what sexual activities transmit HIV and how to avoid infection; and how to obtain and properly use condoms. Among participants who completed the program, awareness of HIV and AIDS increased. Additionally, "completers" were more likely to request condoms for personal use. Similarly, Herman and colleagues (1994) utilized a ten-session intervention that provided information about AIDS, demonstrations of condom use, communication and assertiveness lessons, and techniques for recognizing and managing high risk situations. Posttest evaluations demonstrated satisfactory AIDS knowledge and an intention to change certain high risk behaviors such as unprotected sex and engaging in sexual behavior with strangers.

The third category of HIV prevention strategies for the seriously mentally ill has employed stricter research methods, including randomized designs, control groups, and the use of behavior change as a dependent variable. In addition to education, these programs have attempted to address attitudes and belief systems that contribute to the risky sexual behaviors manifested by a large subset of the seriously mentally ill (Carey et al., 1997). For example, Kalichman and colleagues (1995) randomly assigned 23 participants (11 women) to an HIV prevention program that consisted of four weekly 90-minute sessions and 29 participants (14 women) to a waiting list control group. These sessions provided information on HIV transmission routes, taught risk-reduction strategies such as identifying warning signs that signal sexual risk-producing situations, helped individuals learn how to resist coercive advances by potential sexual partners, and reviewed the benefits and limitations of condom use, as well as the correct application and removal of a condom. The experimental group scored significantly higher on measures of knowledge of condom use and AIDS information than the control group, had significantly stronger intentions to use condoms consistently, and reported significant behavior changes immediately following the interventions, including decreased frequency of unprotected intercourse, and increased frequency and occasions of sexual intercourse during which condoms were used. These behaviors remained improved two months after the intervention. A similar study that utilized a six-session HIV prevention training with single gender groups demonstrated essentially the same positive results (Weinhardt, Carey & Carey, 1997).

In an effort to tease out the essential components of an HIV prevention program for the seriously mentally ill, Kelly (1997) randomly assigned 104 participants into three groups: (1) a one-session risk education control group; (2) a seven-session intervention encompassing general education, skills training, and problem-solving targeted toward risk reduction; and (3) a seven-session intervention that focused on training risk reduction skills as well as teaching participants to communicate their knowledge of AIDS and at-risk behaviors to friends and family members. Knowledge about AIDS, perceived risk-reduction self-efficacy, condom use expectancies, perceived norms regarding safe sex, and a detailed record of sexual behaviors in the past month were measured at baseline and three months after the intervention. Subjects in all three conditions improved in knowledge and belief measures, with a greater magnitude of change in the groups that received the seven-session interventions. The greatest change in sexual behaviors, such as reductions in the number of casual sexual partners and lower rates of unprotected sex, was found in the group given the intervention that included teaching others about AIDS prevention. Similarly, Susser and colleagues (1998) found that their interactive "Sex, Games, and Videotapes" intervention was superior to a passive learning approach for reducing sexual risk behaviors among homeless, mentally ill men.

Although few psychiatric rehabilitation programs have comprehensively addressed the sexual and intimacy needs of the seriously mentally ill, the studies conducted to date have demonstrated the feasibility of their use and the enthusiasm of the participants for the subject matter (Steiner, Lussier, Maust, DiPalma & Allende, 1994). Given the apparent need for this type of material, practitioners' difficulties with expressing sexual material (Withersty, 1976; Coverdale & Aruffo, 1992) can not fully explain the relative rarity of such programs. Perhaps another contributing factor is that many individuals with serious mental illness are deficient in vital areas of social functioning, potentially obscuring from the clinician's view the importance of their sexuality. It is not surprising, therefore, that sexuality issues frequently arise in the context of social skills training, because this modality is geared toward eliciting the goals and desires of participants. As such, skills training technology is a good place to start when constructing a program designed to provide explicit instructions to individuals with serious mental illness in the realms of friendship, dating, intimacy, and sexuality. A brief overview of the modular approach to teaching social skills follows.

Modules for Training Social and Independent Living Skills

Based on the cognitive model of social skills training, a set of psychoeducational modules has been developed at the University of California at Los Angeles (UCLA) Clinical Research Center for Schizophrenia and Psychiatric Rehabilitation (see Table 6.1) with the objectives of (1) teaching patients the social and instrumental competencies of key domains of community functioning, and (2) being easily and accurately used by interdisciplinary professionals and paraprofessionals in a wide array of mental health facilities and natural environments (Liberman *et al.*, 1993). The domains for training these skills include self-management of antipsychotic medication, identifying warning signs of relapse, coping with psychotic symptoms, grooming and personal hygiene, recreation for leisure, interpersonal problem-solving, job finding, community re-entry, family coping, street smarts, and engaging in friendly conversations. Those domains were chosen because competency in them has been associated with better social adjustment, longer community tenure, and lowered risk for relapse and rehospitalization (Liberman, 1992).

Each module uses the same highly structured and thoroughly specified instructional techniques so that professionals can use them with a minimum of training and consultation. The techniques also compensate for patients' cognitive dysfunctions by employing overlearning, visual as well as auditory instruction, and *in vivo* training. Each module is a self-contained package that can be adopted alone or in combination with other modules as part of comprehensive rehabilitation programs.

The training modules have been constructed to teach patients specific functional skills, solve problems that may be encountered while attempting to use newly learned skills, and practice the skills in

Table 6.1. UCLA Social and Independent Living Skills Modules.

Medication Management
Symptom Management
Grooming and Personal Hygiene
Recreation for Leisure
Community Re-Entry
Basic Conversation

the natural environment. This model of social skills training offers considerable promise for those patients who have the cognitive capacity for learning social skills in small groups. Each module is divided into separate skill areas, with each area having specific behaviors that are taught to achieve personal effectiveness and competence. For example, the Medication Management Module contains skills areas for (1) understanding the benefits of antipsychotic medication, (2) acquiring the skills of medication self-administration, (3) coping with the side effects of medication, and (4) negotiating medication issues with health-care providers. Similarly, the Symptom Management Module includes four specific skill areas: (1) identifying the early warning signs of relapse, (2) managing a prodrome and developing a relapse prevention plan, (3) coping with persistent symptoms, and (4) avoiding street drugs and alcohol.

Each module is composed of a prescriptive clinician's manual or guide, a videotape for demonstrating the skills to be learned, and a patient workbook containing practice exercises and monitoring forms. Skills are trained by using a combination of focused instructions, videotaped demonstrations, role-played rehearsals, social and videotaped feedback, problem solving, and practice in the natural environment through *in vivo exercises* and *homework* assignments. Patients proceed through each skill area in a specific sequence of learning exercises and activities, starting with an *Introduction* that aims to highlight the values and advantages of the module. The training procedure emphasizes the "discovery learning" method as opposed to expository or didactic teaching.

The objective of the first learning activity in the module is to help patients identify the goals of the skill area, the consequences that will occur if the goals are achieved, and the steps needed to achieve each goal. In addition, patients learn the relevance of the skill to their personal life. Following the *Introduction*, patients proceed to the second learning activity, *Videotape Questions and Answers*. Patients view videotaped demonstrations of the correct performance of the skills they are about to learn. The tape is periodically stopped and patients are asked questions to assess their attentiveness and comprehension of the information presented in the videotape demonstration. Incorrect answers result in the replay of the videotape and highlighting of the information needed to correctly answer the question when it is repeated.

Next, patients are asked to practice in a *Role Play Exercise* the skills they have just learned. This performance is videotaped for subsequent review by patients and the therapist. The therapist evaluates the performance and provides positive feedback and suggestions for improvement. The role play is then reenacted and the process is repeated until the patient exhibits mastery of the relevant skill.

The next two components, *Resource Management* and *Outcome Problems*, are designed to teach patients methods to overcome the obstacles they may encounter as they attempt to utilize their skills in their natural environment. The training in solving resource management problems is designed to teach patients how to identify and gather the resources necessary to implement a particular skill. Training in solving outcome problems teaches patients how to respond when the environment fails to provide the expected outcome following the performance of a particular skill.

The next two learning activities, *In Vivo Exercises* and *Homework* are used to facilitate the transfer of training from the classroom to the natural environment. In the former, the patient performs the skills outside the classroom accompanied by the skills trainer, who is there to prompt and reinforce the patient's performance, as well as to provide corrective feedback. The latter provides the patient with an opportunity to perform the learned skills independently. Finally, *Booster Sessions* are available on an as-needed basis to maintain skills.

Meta-analyses and reviews of the more than 40 controlled studies of social skills training have shown that individuals with schizophrenia can acquire and retain skills, and that training is associated with significant favorable effects on social adjustment, symptoms, relapse, and rehospitalization rates (Benton & Schroeder, 1990). Recent studies of skills training have shown significant methodological advances including the use of control or comparison groups, increased reliability of assessments, and a better understanding of the cognitive psychology of schizophrenia and the distortions in learning processes commonly encountered (Marder, Wirshing, Mintz, McKenzie, Johnston, Eckman, Lebell, Zimmerman & Liberman, 1996). Further light has been shed on the effectiveness of skills training by way of consistent findings that training leads to diminished symptom levels and improved social and interpersonal skills (Wallace, Liberman, MacKain & Blackwell, 1992). There is strong evidence that skills training leads to skill acquisition and maintenance in schizophrenia, especially if it is intensive (i.e., at least two sessions per week) and of sufficient (i.e., between three and six months) duration (Eckman, Wirshing, Marder, Liberman, Johnston-Cronck, Zimmerman & Mintz, 1992). While schizophrenic patients with even high levels of hallucinations and delusions can acquire skills through systematic training, cognitive disorganization (e.g., severe distractibility and thought disorder) and the deficit syndrome (i.e., primary negative symptoms) appear to markedly interfere with the training process (Kopelowicz, Liberman, Mintz & Zarate, 1997).

The impact and utility of social skills training also can be documented through professional validation; that is, the extent to which the modality is implemented by practitioners and by mental health facilities. The modules for training social and independent living skills, developed at the UCLA Clinical Research Center for Schizophrenia and Psychiatric Rehabilitation, have been implemented in all 50 states by over 1,000 private and public hospitals, community support programs, mental health centers, and practitioners in private practice. A survey of users of the modules found that 61% of the respondents were using the modules regularly, with another 36% planning to institute or reinstitute the modules when administrative and logistical obstacles were overcome (Kopelowicz, Cooper & Liberman, 1995). In addition, the modules have been translated into 15 languages and are in use in Asia, Europe, South America, and Africa. Controlled studies have validated the efficacy of the modules in Quebec, France, Switzerland, Germany, Finland, Bulgaria, Poland and Japan (Liberman, 1998). The growing utilization of skills training methods around the world and their adaptation to local culture and conditions heightens the value of this modality as a major technique in psychiatric rehabilitation. Moreover, the user-friendliness of the method allows for training in even the most complicated of human relations; namely, in the domain of intimacy and sexuality.

Friendship, Dating and Sexuality Module

The Friendship, Dating and Sexuality Module follows the structure of the other modules in the UCLA Social and Independent Living Skills series. This most recent addition to the series uses seven *Skill Areas*, each made up of a distinct body of information and a set of incremental skills that lead participants to the goal of achieving a safe and satisfying sexual relationship (see Table 6.2). The module uses a plot line that follows a couple whose relationship develops from friendship and dating to sexual involvement. In the context of a maturing relationship they demonstrate appropriate communication skills with each other, with trusted friends, and with health care professionals. It is important to note that the module contains sexually explicit material, thus requiring the trainer to be comfortable in discussing intimate sexual issues.

Skill Area I, *Fundamental Knowledge of Sexuality*, introduces the participant to some basic information about sexuality. This skill area includes four vignettes that focus on conception, contraception, sexual desire, and sexually transmitted diseases. In the first vignette, the main

Table 6.2. Skill Areas of the UCLA Friendship, Dating and Sexuality Module.

I. Fundamental Knowledge of Sexuality
II. Sexual Decision-Making
III. Sharing Information with a Partner About Sexuality
IV. Verbal and Nonverbal Skills Before Sex
V. Learning Appropriate Sexual Behavior
VI. Communication Skills After Sexual Intercourse
VII. Sexual Problems: Desire, Arousal and Orgasm

---

characters, Jim and Katie, visit a physician to elicit the information they need prior to including sex in their relationship. They present their concerns to their doctor by explaining, "We've been seeing each other for some time now and we're thinking about having sex. Where do we start? What's important for us to know?" They are led by their physician through an explicit discussion of the risks of engaging in sexual activity. Specific information on a variety of sexually transmitted diseases is provided, including details on the most common diseases, symptoms to look for, and appropriate treatments. Further information is presented on the advantages and disadvantages of various forms of birth control, as well as commonly occurring sexual dysfunctions.

The next vignette features three young people, kin to the main characters, who have their own discussion about contraception and the notion of shared responsibility between partners in a loving relationship. This second vignette reinforces the use of contraception as a means of avoiding unwanted pregnancy and as a way of maintaining good health. Abstinence from sex is also included as a viable option.

The third and fourth vignettes in Skill Area I demonstrate how the knowledge presented earlier can be used in a practical and realistic situation. In the third vignette, Jim goes to a pharmacy to purchase condoms. He is assisted by a pharmacist who reminds him why condoms are recommended, that is, "to prevent pregnancy and to avoid sexually transmitted diseases" and how to shop for condoms, "buy latex only, choose a balloon tip, decide on lubrication." In the fourth vignette, the scene is repeated except that Katie goes to the pharmacy by herself to purchase condoms.

In each of these vignettes, visual aids are used to model important component skills. For example, the physician in the first vignette utilizes a picture of the female reproductive anatomy to help explain the reproductive cycle. Similarly, when contraception is discussed, actual birth control materials are shown as their functions are described. In the third and fourth vignettes, the pharmacist uses a plastic model of an erect penis to demonstrate the correct application of a condom.

The rationale for including Skill Area II, *Sexual Decision-Making*, is that any decision regarding sex is more that just, "Are we going to do it or not?" Rather, sexual decisions can and should be considered in the context of consequences, positive and negative, for either including or not including sex in a loving relationship. Figure 6.1 illustrates the decision matrix that is used throughout this skill area.

Skill Area II follows the protagonists as they discuss the consequences of including or not including sex in a relationship. These conversations elaborate on both the positive and negative aspects of the physical, financial, familial, employment, relationship, and emotional consequences of engaging in sexual behavior. Sexual decision making is demonstrated in seven vignettes, including conversations between two male friends, two female friends, a couple in a serious relationship

	POSITIVE CONSEQUENCES	NEGATIVE CONSEQUENCES
AFFIRM:	1. _____	1. _____
[Decision to	2. _____	2. _____
engage in	3. _____	3. _____
sexual behavior]	4. _____	4. _____
REJECT:	1. _____	1. _____
[Decision to	2. _____	2. _____
not engage in	3. _____	3. _____
sexual behavior]	4. _____	4. _____

Figure 6.1. Basic Decision Matrix.

(Jim and Katie) and between them and a second couple who have a young child. The opening scene occurs as two men discuss the physical consequences of having versus not having sex. They cover a variety of areas in a conversation that ranges from, "Nothing feels better than making love," and "With the right person I might want to have a baby" to "I might not get an erection," and "What would happen if one of us has a sexually-transmitted disease?" Figure 6.2 illustrates the model in which physical consequences of having/not having sex are presented.

A conversation between two women illustrates the potential familial and employment consequences of including sex in relationships. Positive consequences include, "My parents would love to have grandchildren," and "My last boss thinks people work better if they are in a relationship." Negative consequences include, "His parents might think I took advantage of their son" and "We almost got fired because we got caught grabbing and touching each other." Figure 6.3 illustrates the decision matrix that generates a discussion of familial consequences of including/not including sex in a relationship.

Relationship and emotional consequences of having/not having sex are modeled by Jim and Katie. They mutually acknowledge that they are in a committed relationship and that they have been thinking about becoming sexual with each other. Two vignettes show them discussing the potential consequences of adding or not adding sex to their relationship. Their conversation includes statements such as, "If we start having sex, we'll be more sure about our love for each other," and, "I would feel even more committed to you." Negative consequences are presented as well. For example, "We might lose the great relationship we already have." Figure 6.4 illustrates the matrix that is used to generate decision making around emotional consequences.

The final vignette in this skill area places sexual decision making in a real-life context as an unmarried couple discusses the consequences

POSITIVE CONSEQUENCES	NEGATIVE CONSEQUENCES
1. Orgasm (feels good)	1. AIDS or other STDs
2. Relaxing	2. Painful
AFFIRM 3. Physically Comforting	3. Physical Frustration/Tension
4. Pregnancy	4. Pregnancy
5. Acquire Skills	5. Fatigue
1. Relaxation of Tension	1. Tension
REJECT 2. No Unwanted Pregnancy	2. No Wanted Pregnancy
3. Avoids AIDS or STDs	3. Lack of Physical Closeness
	4. No Acquisition of Skills

Figure 6.2. Physical Consequences of Engaging or Not Engaging in Sexual Behavior.

of having a child whom they both love, but who was not planned. The parents discuss, and at times argue about, the pressures they face. From losing sleep, having to take a second job, and lack of support from the baby's grandparents, to relapse of psychiatric symptoms and increased alcohol use by one of the parents, both acknowledge that "having sex just one time without a condom" can have significant adverse consequences.

Skill Area III, *Sharing Information with a Partner About Sexuality*, introduces the very contemporary and vitally important topic of giving and eliciting a sexual history from a partner. Jim and Katie exchange information about their previous sexual contacts. Emphasis is placed on self-disclosure, particularly with respect to past and current partners, and the recognition that one cannot safely assume the absence of sexually transmitted disease because of a current lack of symptoms. Jim and Katie acknowledge that they are both willing to be tested for sexually transmitted diseases and agree to make their relationship monogamous.

The next skill area, *Verbal and Nonverbal Skills Before Sex*, introduces an essential set of communication skills. These so-called "**Go/No Go**" signals include the subtle and not so subtle cues that people use to indicate interest in a two-way conversation or an exchange of information. In this module, **Go/No Go** signals are used by the couple to

POSITIVE CONSEQUENCES	NEGATIVE CONSEQUENCES
1. Have Own Family	1. Creation of Own Family When Not Ready
2. Improve Family Relations	2. Family Relations May Deteriorate
AFFIRM 3. Perpetuation of Family	3. Displacement
	4. Denying Other Problems
1. Trust	1. Pressure from Parents and
2. Respect from Couples' Parents	Friends to Procreate
REJECT 3. Kids Won't Witness	2. Feelings of Rejection from Parents
4. No Unwanted Children	3. Absence of Closeness with Parents
	4. Acrimony/Power Struggle with Parents

Figure 6.3. Familial Consequences of Engaging or Not Engaging in Sexual Behavior.

communicate a lack of interest in pursuing sexual activity or to reinforce a partner's sexual advances. Acquiring the skill to accurately read a partner's **Go/No Go** signals is a prerequisite to good communication and to achieving a satisfying sexual relationship.

This skill area uses nine brief vignettes to model nonverbal and verbal communication related to sexual activity. All vignettes involve interactions between Jim and Katie as they demonstrate the following activities: nonverbal **No Go** behavior, for example, lack of eye contact, yawning, body orientation; **No Go** verbal signals, for example, "No dear, I'm not in the mood tonight"; non-verbal **Go** signals, for example, eye contact, smiles, reciprocating touches; and, verbal **Go** signals, for example, "My day just got better now that you're here."

In addition to a thorough modeling of **Go/No Go** signals, Skill Area IV also includes a review of sexual decision making and emphasizes the setting of limits as important preludes to engaging in sexual behavior. Jim and Katie are seen engaged in passionate kissing, behavior that may lead to sexual intercourse. The limit setting behavior that is modeled includes a statement, "Not tonight, I'm too tired. How about just hugging and kissing?" A reasonable response is also observed, "That's fine with me." Other vignettes include other possible scenarios, such

POSITIVE CONSEQUENCES	NEGATIVE CONSEQUENCES
1. Love	1. Regret
2. Happiness	2. Guilt/shame
AFFIRM 3. Fulfillment	3. Loss of Self-respect
4. Health, Normality, Self-esteem	4. Confusion
5. Increased Commitment	5. Feelings of Incompetence
6. Security	6. Disappointment with Partner
1. Pride in Health Self-Control	1. Frustration
2. Self-Respect	2. Anger
REJECT 3. Increased Love, Respect	3. Sadness
	4. Insecurity
	5. Regret
	6. Feeling Defective ("What's Wrong With Me?")
	7. Confusion

Figure 6.4. Emotional Consequences of Engaging or Not Engaging in Sexual Behavior.

as, "Let's not have intercourse tonight. We could stimulate each other and have an orgasm without intercourse." In addition, limit setting is modeled when Jim and Katie discover that neither one of them has condoms. The last vignette of this skill area sets the stage for sexual intercourse. Jim and Katie are alone, they have committed to a monogamous relationship with each other, they have made a well-reasoned decision about having sex, they have been tested for sexually transmitted diseases, and they have a supply of condoms. They are thus ready for the next step.

In Skill Area V, *Learning Appropriate Sexual Behavior*, a range of sexual behaviors are modeled. These include appropriate touching, communication skills preceding sexual relationships, for example, asking permission, and communication skills while engaged in a sexual encounter, such as attending to the needs of your partner. Limit setting and respectful compliance is demonstrated in the opening vignette. A simple request is made, "Please don't touch me like that in public," followed by, "I understand." A second brief vignette simply models how to come to an agreement on the time and place for being together to engage in sexual intercourse.

The vignettes that follow all include full nudity. To desensitize viewers, Katie and Jim are first seen nude individually, at their own apartments, preparing for the date that will culminate in their first sexual encounter. As they look at their bodies in the mirror just after showering, Katie thinks aloud, "I wonder if I'll be able to tell him how I like to be touched?" Jim thinks aloud, "I wonder if I'll be able to guide Katie in the way I like to be touched." The vignette ends with Jim remembering to bring latex condoms as he leaves for his rendezvous with Katie.

In the next few vignettes, explicit sexual behavior, including intercourse, is graphically depicted. Jim and Katie meet in their friend's apartment. They acknowledge both their eagerness for sexual intercourse and their nervousness about adding that new dimension to their relationship. Katie states her interest in not moving ahead too fast, "I brought some massage oil. Why don't we start with a backrub?" Jim demonstrates how to ask permission before he moves on, "Can I unhook your bra?" Limit setting and a request for behavior is modeled, "I'm not ready for you to lie on top of me. I'll massage you before we put on the condom. Is that okay?" A "guided hands" technique is presented as Katie shows Jim how to massage her breasts and in turn, Jim guides Katie's hands in stroking his penis. Safe and appropriate use of a condom and spermicidal jelly is modeled as this series of vignettes is concluded.

The final vignette of this skill area focuses on Jim and Katie after their sexual relationship has matured for a few months. They acknowledge their initial awkwardness and the importance of communicating their sexual needs. This skill area closes with a sexual encounter that "puts it all together" as Jim and Katie demonstrate the skills they have learned. The component skills (giving and receiving permission, assertive requests, guided hands) are combined into a free-flowing, loving, and tender sexual encounter.

Skill Area VI, *Communication Skills After Sexual Intercourse*, involves two brief vignettes. In both, Jim and Katie engage in appropriate verbal and nonverbal communication after they have had intercourse. They mutually reinforce each other for their decision making, for being able to give specific instructions about how they like to be touched, and for pleasing each other.

Skill Area VII, *Sexual Problems: Desire, Arousal, and Orgasm*, uses a number of vignettes to present common problems related to the phases of sexual response; namely, desire, arousal, and orgasm. The purpose for including this section is to provide education about sexual functioning, normalize problems of desire, arousal, and orgasm, and to teach effective problem solving methods when sexual dysfunctions occur. Vignettes include scenes of Jim and Katie talking with their respective male and female friends/confidants, and Jim and Katie alone.

Problems of sexual desire are discussed when Jim meets with his friend Jake and they exchange personal information about sexual experiences. Jim raises the subject, "Katie and I went out last night and saw a good movie. After that we went to her place and I could tell she was in the mood for making love. But, I just didn't have any desire to have sex. Is there something wrong with me?" Jake assures Jim that lack of desire for sex occurs normally and that there is usually a simple explanation for why desire is low, for example, fatigue, illness, worry, or preoccupation about other matters.

Jim and Katie confront lack of sexual desire in their relationship and they model a reasonable response when Jim states, "I don't really want to make love tonight." They are able to admit that they have each felt a lack of sexual desire, "When I'm tired or if I am getting over being sick." Further, they demonstrate continued affection and support for each other without insistence on sexual intercourse whenever they are together.

Katie seeks advice about her lack of sexual arousal when she visits with her friend, Mary. She states, "Jim was touching my breasts and that usually turns me on. But, not last night. Is there something wrong with me?" Mary assures Katie that sexual arousal is not automatic, occasional lack of arousal is normal and that she can probably find an explanation for not becoming aroused. Mary asks, "Are you taking any medication? A side effect of some medications is that you are less able to become aroused."

Katie and Jim reenact the scenario when they are in bed together. Their behavior initially suggests that they both desire to have sex but Katie soon stops and states, "I'm in the mood to make love, but I'm just not getting turned on. I think that it might be my medication." She and Jim discuss how the problem might be solved, "I'll talk to my doctor. Maybe he can give me a medication that doesn't have that side effect." Katie also suggests options to intercourse, "I can stimulate you in other ways. It's okay if you don't try to turn me on. We could just snuggle."

Additional sexual arousal problems, such as the lack of an erection, and factors that effect arousal, are presented in several interspersed vignettes. Emotional and relationship concerns are raised as Jim and Katie acknowledge occasional anxiety and worry. For example, Katie states, "I'm afraid of falling deeper in love. I might really get hurt. I wanted to make love but I just got scared. What if Jim tells me he's not really in love with me?"

This skill area also provides information about dysfunctions of the orgasm phase of sexual response, including absence of orgasm, rapid ejaculation, delayed ejaculation, and painful intercourse. As above, vignettes involving Jim and his friend Jake, and Katie and her friend Mary, are interspersed with scenes where Jim and Katie are in bed together. Mary assures Katie, "If you're not feeling well or are upset about something you might not have an orgasm. Maybe it would help if you show Jim exactly how and where you want to be touched. It's normal to not have an orgasm every time you make love." Jim and Katie assure each other that they are able to enjoy being sexual with each other without insisting on having an orgasm.

CONCLUSIONS

A number of caveats must be considered by professionals who wish to use the Friendship, Dating, and Sexuality module. First, prior to conducting groups with patients, staff must be trained in a manner similar to the one used with other modules in the UCLA Social and Independent Living Skills series. This training takes place in a group setting, with staff members assuming the roles of trainers, co-trainers, and participants. Each learning activity is practiced until mastery, confidence, and comfort is achieved. Second, trainers must familiarize themselves with the content and structure of the module. To compensate for patients' attentional and cognitive difficulties, the material is presented in a graphic manner. As such, trainers will need to desensitize themselves to the visually explicit sexual nature of the module.

Another reason for trainers to become familiar with the module prior to conducting a group is that they can pick and choose the segments that are most appropriate for their clients. For example, some clients may benefit from the module's didactic material such as education regarding contraception, conception, and sexually transmitted diseases in Skill Area I, while others may wish to focus on the friendship and dating skill areas. Both of these types of clients could participate in the group and yet avoid the more explicit material presented in the later skill areas. Nevertheless, trainers should recognize that clients' psychiatric symptoms may be sensitive to the explicit nature of the emotional and sexual content of the module, even in skill areas that may seem "tame." Therefore, trainers must monitor clients' reactions and assist clients with monitoring their symptoms. A problem solving exercise is recommended if a deterioration of symptoms occurs. Usually, "cooling off" breaks are sufficient when explicit material is presented, but participants also can be reminded to use symptom management strategies, or even to discuss the possibility of medication changes with their psychiatrist if necessary.

Additionally, professionals who supervise skills trainers, and trainers themselves, should be aware of emerging medical and psychological research regarding sexuality. Human sexuality, sexually transmitted diseases, and disease prevention are all dynamic fields of investigation and new research may affect the material presented in the module. For example, findings on the lack of effectiveness of spermicidal cream with nonyxonol-9 for preventing HIV transmission was announced after the taping of the module's video was completed. This data necessitated the re-taping of a portion of the video incorporating this vitally important information. Similarly, trainers will need to keep abreast of research findings to provide accurate information to group members.

In summary, the theme of this chapter has been the need to provide individuals coping with serious mental illness with the skills required to enter into and nurture a mutually respectful, loving relationship. It is important for clinicians to remember that this task is consistent with the most basic goals of psychiatric rehabilitation; namely, the optimization of psychosocial performance, community re-integration, and quality of life improvement. An individual with serious mental illness enjoying such relationships, which oftentimes may incorporate safe and satisfying sex, should be recognized by clinicians, family members, and society at large as taking an empowering, healthy, and productive step on the road to sustained recovery.

REFERENCES

Akhtar, S. & Thomson, J.A. (1980). Schizophrenia and sexuality: A review and a report of twelve unusual cases. *Journal of Clinical Psychiatry* 41:134–142.

Benton, M.K. & Schroeder, H.E. (1990). Social skills training with schizophrenics: A meta-analytic evaluation. *Journal of Consulting and Clinical Psychology* 58:741–747.

Brady, S.M. & Carmen, E. (1990). AIDS risk in the chronically mentally ill: Clinical strategies for prevention. *New Directions for Mental Health Services* 48:83–95.

Carey, M.P., Weinhardt, L.S. & Carey, K.B. (1995). Prevalence of infection with HIV among the seriously mentally ill: Review of research and implications for practice. *Professional Psychology: Research and Practice* 26: 262–268.

Carey, M.P., Carey, K.B., Weinhardt, L.S. & Gordon C.M. (1997). Behavioral risk for HIV infection among adults with a severe and persistent mental illness: Patterns and psychological antecedents. *Community Mental Health Journal* 33:133–141.

Coverdale, J.H. & Aruffo, J. (1992). AIDS and family planning counseling of psychiatrically ill women in community mental health clinics. *Community Mental Health Journal* 28:13–20.

Davidhizar, R., Boonstra, C., Lutz, K. & Poston, P. (1991). Teaching safer sex in a long-term psychiatric setting. *Perspectives in Psychiatric Care* 27: 25–29.

Eckman, T.A., Wirshing, W.C., Marder, S.R., Liberman, R.P., Johnston-Cronk, K., Zimmerman, K. & Mintz, J. (1992). Techniques for training schizophrenic patients in illness self-management: A controlled trial. *American Journal of Psychiatry* 149:1549–1555.

Friedman, M. (1976). Family life-sex education as an adjunct to psychiatric treatment. *The Family Coordinator* 24:297–302.

Friedman, S. & Harrison, G. (1984). Sexual histories, attitudes, and behavior of schizophrenic and "normal" women. *Archives of Sexual Behavior* 13:555–567.

Goisman, R.M., Kent, A.B., Montgomery, E.C., Cheevers, M.M. & Goldfinger S.M. (1991). AIDS education for patients with chronic mental illness. *Community Mental Health Journal* 27:189–197.

Graham, L.L. & Cates, J.A. (1992). To reduce the risk of HIV infection for the mentally ill. *Journal of Psychosocial Nursing* 30:9–13.

Herman, R., Kaplan, M., Satriano, J., Cournos, F. & McKinnon, K. (1994). HIV prevention with people with serious mental illness: Staff training and institutional attitudes. *Psychosocial Rehabilitation Journal* 17:98–103.

Howden, M., Zipple, A.M. & Tyrrell, W.F. (1994). Dating skills for residential consumers. *Psychosocial Rehabilitation Journal* 18:67–74.

Jones, T.R. (1983). Treatment approaches to sexual problems with dual diagnosis clients. *Journal of Social Work and Human Sexuality* 2:113–130.

Kalichman, S.C., Sikkema, K.J., Kelly, J.A. & Bulto, M. (1995). Use of a brief behavioral skills intervention to prevent HIV infection among chronic mentally ill adults. *Psychiatric Services* 46:275–280.

Kalichman, S.C., Carey, M.P. & Carey, K.B. (1996). Human immuodeficiency virus (HIV) risk among the seriously mentally ill. *Clinical Psychology: Science and Practice* 3:130–143.

Kelly, J.A. (1997). HIV risk reduction interventions for persons with severe mental illness. *Clinical Psychology Review* 17:293–309.

Kopelowicz (1994). Friendship, intimacy and sexuality. *The Journal of the California Alliance for the Mentally Ill* 5 (1):7–8.

Kopelowicz, A. & Liberman, R.P. (1994). Self-management approaches for seriously mentally ill persons. *Directions in Psychiatry* 14 (17):1–8.

Kopelowicz, A., Cooper, L. & Liberman, R.P. (1995). Social skills training and psychiatric rehabilitation. *World Association of Psychiatric Rehabilitation Bulletin* 7:6–7.

Kopelowicz, A., Corrigan, P., Wallace, C. & Liberman, R.P. (1996). Biopsychosocial rehabilitation. In Tasman, A., Kay, J. & Lieberman, J.A. (Eds.): *Psychiatry* (pp. 1513–1534). Philadelphia: W.B. Saunders Company.

Kopelowicz, A., Liberman, R.P., Mintz, J. & Zarate, R. (1997). Efficacy of social skills training for deficit versus nondeficit negative symptoms in schizophrenia. *American Journal of Psychiatry* 154:424–425.

Laumann, E.O., Gagnon, J.H., Michael, R.T. & Michaels, S. (1994). *The Social Organization of Sexuality.* Chicago: University of Chicago Press.

Liberman, R.P. (1992). *Handbook of Psychiatric Rehabilitation.* Boston: Allyn and Bacon.

Liberman, R.P., Wallace, C.J., Blackwell, G., Eckman, T.A., Vaccaro, J.V. & Kuehnel, T.G. (1993). Innovations in skills training for the seriously mentally ill: The UCLA Social and Independent Living Skills modules. *Innovations and Research* 2:43–60.

Liberman, R.P. (1998). International utilization of the UCLA Social and Independent Living Skills modules. *International Review of Psychiatry* 10:1–14.

Lukoff, D., Gioia-Hasick, D., Sullivan, G., Golden, J.S. & Nuechterlein, K.H. (1986). Sex education and rehabilitation with schizophrenic male outpatients. *Schizophrenia Bulletin* 12:669–676.

Marder, S.R., Wirshing, W.C., Mintz, J., McKenzie, J., Johnston, K., Eckman, T.A., Lebell, M., Zimmerman, K. & Liberman, R.P. (1996). Two-year outcome of social skills training and group psychotherapy for outpatients with schizophrenia. *American Journal of Psychiatry* 153:1585–1592.

McEvoy, J.P., Hatcher, A., Applebaum, P.S. & Abernethy, V. (1993). Chronic schizophrenic women's attitudes toward sex, pregnancy, birth control, and childrearing. *Hospital and Community Psychiatry* 34:536–539.

Pinderhughes, C.A., Grace, E.B. & Reyna, L.J. (1972). Psychiatric disorders and sexual functioning. *American Journal of Psychiatry* 128:1276–1283.

Steiner, J.L., Lussier, R.G., Maust, G.C., DiPalma, L.M. & Allende, M.J. (1994). Psychoeducation about sexual issues in an acute treatment setting. *Hospital and Community Psychiatry* 45:380–381.

Susser, E., Valencia, E., Berkman, A., Sohler, N., Conover, S., Torres, J., Betne, P., Felix, A. & Miller, S. (1998). Human Immunodeficiency Virus Sexual

Risk Reduction in Homeless Men with Mental Illness. *Archives of General Psychiatry* 55:266–272.

Uttaro, T. & Mechanic, D. (1994). The NAMI consumer survey analysis of unmet needs. *Hospital and Community Psychiatry* 45:372–374.

Wallace, C.J., Liberman, R.P., MacKain, S.J. & Blackwell, G. (1992). Effectiveness and replicability of modules for teaching social and instrumental skills to the severely mentally ill. *American Journal of Psychiatry* 149:654–658.

Wasow, M. (1980). Sexuality and the institutionalized mentally ill. *Sexuality and Disability* 3:3–16.

Weiden, P., Aquila, R. & Standard, J. (1996). Atypical antipsychotic drugs and long-term outcome of schizophrenia. *Journal of Clinical Psychiatry* 57 (11): 53–60.

Weinhardt, L.W., Carey, M.P. & Carey, K.B. (1997). HIV risk reduction for the seriously mentally ill: Pilot investigation and call for research. *Journal of Behavior Therapy and Experimental Psychiatry* 28:87–95.

Withersty, D.J. (1976). Sexual attitudes of hospital personnel: A model for continuing education. *American Journal of Psychiatry* 133:573–575.

7

HIV and Serious Mental Illness

KAREN McKINNON and
FRANCINE COURNOS

Infection with human immunodeficiency virus (HIV) has been documented in one in 12 adults in treatment for serious mental illness in areas of the United States where seroprevalence studies have been conducted (Cournos & McKinnon, 1997). Understanding what has fueled the spread of HIV in this population can help mental health care providers to recognize when their patients are at risk for acquiring or transmitting the virus. People in treatment for severe psychiatric disorders often depend on mental health staff for referrals to appropriate medical care, and clinicians in psychiatric settings are increasingly called upon to help their clients make HIV-related testing and treatment decisions. This chapter presents an overview of the complex HIV-related issues involved.

THE SCOPE OF THE AIDS EPIDEMIC AMONG PEOPLE WITH SERIOUS MENTAL ILLNESS IN THE UNITED STATES

HIV first appeared in the United States in 1978 (Conant, 1984), and the virus spread unchecked for several years before being identified. The first published reports of AIDS cases among adults in psychiatric hospitals and clinics only appeared in the late 1980s (e.g., Gewirtz, Horwath, Cournos & Empfield, 1988). The scarcity of prevalence data about the sexual and drug-using behaviors of adults with serious mental illness slowed the design of usable AIDS prevention interventions for psychiatric patients (Auerbach, Wypijewska & Brodie, 1994), allowing the virus to spread without impediment well into the 1990s.

Prevalence of HIV Infection

A dozen studies of HIV infection among people with serious mental illness have been published to date and yield a combined seroprevalence of 7.8% (Cournos & McKinnon, 1997). All studies in the peer-reviewed literature were conducted in the Northeast, primarily on inpatient units, and may not reflect the epidemic in other regions and populations. Nonetheless, these data are impressive when compared to the estimated HIV infection rate in the general U.S. population for the corresponding period of 0.4% (Steele, 1994).

Rates of HIV infection vary by treatment setting, reflecting the specialized needs of the patients being treated. Infection rates are highest among patients on units that treat comorbid psychiatric and substance (alcohol or other drug) use disorders, where 18.4% of patients were HIV-positive (Lee, Travin & Bluestone, 1992; Silberstein, Galanter, Marmor, Lifshutz & Krasinski, 1994). On these units, positive antibody test results were found among 33.8% of drug injectors, 15.4% of noninjection drug users, 10.9% of alcohol users, and 2.6% of substance users who did not meet criteria for current abuse or dependence diagnoses. Homeless patients had an overall infection rate of 8.5% (Empfield et al., 1993; Meyer, Cournos et al., 1993; Susser, Valencia & Conover, 1993). Rates were higher among patients living in a homeless shelter than among those living on a specialized inpatient ward. The rate of infection among new admissions to psychiatric units was 7.5% (Cournos et al., 1991; Sacks, Dermatis, Looser-Ott, Perry, 1992; Stewart, Zuckerman & Ingle, 1994; Volavka et al., 1991). In the only study of forensic patients, pre-trial detainees had an infection rate of 5.5% (Schwartz-Watts, Montgomery & Morgan, 1995). The lowest rate of HIV infection was found on a long-stay psychiatric unit, where 4.0% of patients were infected (Meyer, McKinnon et al., 1993).

Although seroprevalence data for psychiatric patients are largely drawn from East Coast cities, HIV has been moving from urban epicenters to suburban and rural communities for some time (Cournos, Herman, Kaplan & McKinnon, 1997), so regional differences are shrinking. In one longitudinal study, HIV/AIDS was the leading cause of death among a semi-rural group of young patients in New York state who were experiencing their first psychiatric hospitalization for a psychotic episode (Susser, Colson et al., 1997).

Age and ethnic distributions of HIV infection among psychiatric patients do not differ from the patterns of infection in nonpsychiatric groups, but women with serious mental illness are as likely as their male counterparts to be HIV infected. This gender parity is not yet found in the general population in the U.S., although rates of HIV infection are now increasing fastest among young women who acquire the infection through heterosexual contact (Wortley & Fleming, 1997).

Prevalence of HIV-Related Risk Behaviors

The AIDS epidemic among adults with serious mental illness is fueled by frequent unprotected sexual behaviors, the drug use that fosters them, and, to a significant extent, by drug injection.

Drug injection: HIV can be directly introduced into the bloodstream by injection when needles, other injection equipment, or rinse water contain the blood of an infected drug injector and are then used by another drug injector. When sterile needles and syringes cannot be obtained, bleach can be used to inactivate HIV in injection equipment.

Little is known about drug injection and equipment sharing among people with serious mental illness, and their equipment cleaning practices are entirely unexplored. Injection in the past three to 12 months has been reported by one percent to eight percent of psychiatric patients (Carey, Kalichman, 1997) and prior injection by five percent to 26 percent (Carey et al., 1997; Susser, Miller et al., 1997). Because psychiatric patients who inject tend to do so intermittently rather than regularly, drug injection histories are often missed in mental health settings. However, reinitiation of drug injection has been found to occur among 70% of drug users in the general population who injected in the past one to five years (van Ameijden, van den Hoek, Jartgers & Coutinho, 1994), and the same may be true for people with serious mental illness. Sharing needles or other injection paraphernalia in the past year to five years has been reported by one in 20 psychiatric patients (Susser, Miller et al., 1997), so the likelihood is high that a subset of people with serious mental illness is at risk of exposure to HIV through contaminated injection paraphernalia.

Sexual behavior: Any sexual behavior is risky if it increases the chances of coming in contact with the AIDS virus or susceptibility to infection. HIV can be transmitted during anal, penile-vaginal, and oral-genital intercourse, and sex with people in identified risk groups (e.g., injection drug users) is considered risky because HIV is highly concentrated in these populations. Tissue compromises, such as those that can result from frequent sexual activity or from sexually transmitted diseases, can increase susceptibility to infection with HIV.

Sexual risk behaviors among people in psychiatric treatment are common (Carey et al., 1997). One-half to two-thirds of patients were sexually active with a partner in the past year. Although periodic same-sex intercourse is not atypical in portions of the general population (Laumann, Gagnon, Michael & Michaels, 1994), psychiatric patients appear to engage in same-sex activity more frequently than non-psychiatric groups (Lyketsos, Sakka & Mailis, 1983; Lukianowicz, 1963; Verhulst & Schneidman, 1981; Klaf & Davis, 1960; Lukoff, Gioia-Hasiok, Sullivan, Golden & Neuchterlein, 1986; McDermott, Sautter, Winstead & Quirk, 1994). This may be particularly true of men versus women (Akhtar & Thomson, 1980; Klaf, 1961), which is noteworthy because male same-sex activity confers more HIV risk than female same-sex activity. Same-sex activity within the past year among people with psychiatric disorders ranges from two percent to 30% of men (Carey et al., 1997), and three percent to eight percent of women (Carey et al., 1997). Between one-tenth and one-third of both men and women reported a lifetime history of homosexual behavior (Carey et al., 1997). Multiple sex partners are common among sexually active psychiatric patients. One-third to one-half of sexually active psychiatric inpatients and outpatients, including those with comorbid substance use diagnoses, reported multiple sex partners in the past year (Carey et al., 1997). Women were significantly less likely than men to have multiple sex partners in one sample of acutely ill psychiatric inpatients (Menon & Pomerantz, 1997) but gender differences in having multiple sex partners were not found in other patient groups (Cournos et al., 1994; Kalichman, Kelly, Johnson & Bulto, 1994). Receptive anal intercourse was also more common among women than men in one study (Menon & Pomerantz, 1997) but not in others (Cournos et al., 1994).

There is troubling evidence that the sexual activity of people with serious mental illness is characterized by a lack of condom use in a majority of sexual occasions (Carey et al., 1997). Forty percent of outpatients reported engaging in unprotected vaginal intercourse at least once in the past month (Stevenson et al., 1993). More than half of sexually active inpatients and outpatients, including those with comorbid substance use disorders, reported never using condoms in the past six to 12 months (Hanson et al., 1992; Cournos, McKinnon, Meyer-Bahlburg, Guido & Meyer, 1993). Interestingly, one study found a 50% rate of condom use among psychiatric patients comparable to that of a nonpsychiatric control group (McDermott et al., 1994), which suggests that psychiatric patients may not differ from others in this respect. In fact, a few studies have found consistent condom use for recent sexual activity among eight percent to 25% of sexually active patients (Carey et al., 1997), and one study showed that patients with multiple sex partners reported more condom use in the past six months than patients who had just one sex partner (Cournos et al., 1993). Still, a sizeable group of psychiatric patients is not using condoms commensurate with their risk behavior. For example, 13% of inpatients reported never using condoms with five or more opposite-sex partners over a five-year period (Sacks, Perry, Graver, Shindledecker & Hall, 1990). Gender differences in condom use have not been found.

Co-occurring sexual behavior and drug use: Alcohol and other drugs are thought to contribute to HIV risk by increasing sexual desire, disinhibiting sexual behavior, and interfering with the practice of safer sex. Transmission of HIV often occurs during sexual contact of previously uninfected people with infected drug injectors, although drug injectors may be more likely than the general population to use condoms (Siegel & Gibson, 1988; McKeganey, Barnard & Watson, 1989), and have been found to do so specifically with non drug-using sexual partners (Metsch, 1995).

Many sexually active psychiatric patients report that alcohol or drugs are part of their sexual experience. Among sexually active inpatients and outpatients, 15% to 45% reported using substances during sex in the past six to 12 months (Carey et al., 1997; Menon & Pomerantz, 1997); rates were comparable for men and women. Trading sex for drugs or for money to buy drugs appears to be a common practice among certain people with serious mental illness. Sex exchange within the past year was reported by 13% to 50% of sexually active inpatients and outpatients, 12% of sexually active dual-diagnosis patients, and 47% to 69% of sexually active homeless men receiving psychiatric treatment in a shelter (Carey et al., 1997). Gender may influence who trades drugs for sex and who trades sex for drugs (Morningstar & Chitwood, 1987), but both activities confer risk and may mutually reinforce unsafe sexual behaviors. Unprotected sex with an infected drug injector was reported by three percent to 13% of psychiatric inpatients and outpatients in the past one to twelve months to (Carey et al., 1997). Lifetime prevalence of sex with a drug injector was six percent to nine percent among psychiatric outpatients (Carey et al., 1997). Some patients have sex partners whom they know are HIV-infected. Among inpatients, two percent reported having unprotected sexual activity with a known HIV-positive partner in the past five years, and among outpatients, eight percent of men and four percent of women had sex with a partner with HIV infection, a statistically nonsignificant difference (Carey et al., 1997). Of course in many instances the partner's HIV status is unknown to the patient. Gender differences in the likelihood of having sex with a partner with AIDS have yet to be carefully examined.

The direct link between use of specific substances and unprotected sex has been examined among acute psychiatric inpatients, and a significant association was found for women between using alcohol before or during sex and receptive anal sex, and for men between using crack during sex and two risk behaviors: sex with a high-risk partner and inconsistent condom use (Menon & Pomerantz, 1997). Similar associations between substance use during sex and unsafe sexual behaviors have been reported among gay men (Stall, McKusick & Wiley, 1986) and in the general population (Leigh, 1990). One encouraging finding is that some people with serious mental illness who engage in drug-related sexual risk behaviors are taking steps to protect themselves from exposure. Among patients with comorbid psychiatric and cocaine use disorders, condom use was reported more frequently by patients with the most sexual partners (Kim, Galanter, Castaneda, Lifshutz & Franco, 1992).

Prevalence of Sexually Transmitted Diseases

Having a current or prior sexually transmitted disease (STD) not only indicates unprotected sexual activity but can increase the risk of HIV transmission if there are openings in the skin or mucous membranes. Between nine percent and 33% of psychiatric inpatients and outpatients were diagnosed with one or more STDs at some time in their lives (Carey et al., 1997). One study found that three percent of outpatients reported a sexually transmitted infection in the past year, yet six percent reported having a genital ulceration during the same period (Carey et al., 1997), suggesting that some patients may have STDs without being aware of them.

Determinants of HIV Risk Behaviors

Certain psychiatric features such as cognitive impairment have been assumed to increase HIV risk among people with the most serious and persistent psychiatric disorders, either by directly affecting behavior or by mediating behavior by their effect on the ability to use information about AIDS to engage in safer behaviors. However, little research has attempted to disentangle the complex connections between these factors. Moreover, risk behaviors among people with serious mental illness have been examined almost exclusively from an individual perspective but may be the result of transactions between psychiatric patients, other people affected by HIV, and the social-contextual environments in which people take risks. Even among people who are well informed about AIDS, unsafe behaviors may be difficult to change in the face of competing contingencies and difficult living conditions. Cultural, social, ethnic, and other factors may exert critical influences on sexual and drug use risk behaviors and safer practices.

AIDS knowledge: Knowledge alone has not been shown to reduce risk behaviors, but it is a necessary condition for any health behavior change (Kelly, 1997). In fact, AIDS knowledge among psychiatric patients appears to be relatively good. In studies of a variety of psychiatric patient groups, correct responses to AIDS knowledge questionnaires ranged from 70% to 80% (McKinnon, Cournos, Sugden, Guido & Herman, 1996), a comparable accuracy rate to that found in the general population (Hardy, 1990).

Psychiatric factors that increase risk: Psychiatric symptoms and disabilities are what differentiate this population from others, but clinical observations that certain psychiatric syndromes and risk behaviors are linked have rarely been tested. The few studies that have examined diagnostic differences in sexual activity and abstinence have found either no relationship between diagnosis and being sexually active or, contrary to expectations, an association between being sexually active and schizophrenia but not bipolar disorder (McKinnon *et al.*, 1996). Alcohol use during sex was more common among people with depressive disorders than those with schizophrenia or mania (Menon & Pomerantz, 1997). Bipolar disorder was related to having a drug-injecting sex partner in one study, but only among women, and this association has not been found consistently (McKinnon *et al.*, 1996).

Simultaneous examination of the effects of several specific psychiatric symptom clusters (measured by the Positive and Negative Syndrome Scale) on particular risk behaviors showed that having multiple sex partners was nearly three times as likely among patients with greater positive symptoms of psychosis. Trading sex was more than three times as likely among patients with schizophrenia than among those with other diagnoses and more than five times as likely among those with more excitement symptoms (McKinnon *et al.*, 1996).

The link between psychiatric factors, use of specific substances, and the number of sex partners has been examined in one small study (Hanson *et al.*, 1992) among patients with comorbid psychiatric and cocaine use disorders; those with mood disorders had significantly more sex partners than those with schizophrenia. This study also found that even though sexual desire decreased with prolonged crack use, the number of sexual partners did not necessarily decrease and in many cases increased. Women in this study were more sexually active than men, many of whom were impotent while using crack. However, these men frequently continued to be sexually active, engaging in oral sex.

The link between psychiatric diagnosis and illicit drug injection remains unclear. In one study (McDermott *et al.*, 1994), psychiatric patients had much higher rates of injection in the past five years than a nonpsychiatric control group. This study also found differences within the psychiatric patient group: injection was significantly more common among those with depressive disorder than those with schizophrenia, and patients with bipolar disorder had the lowest rates of all. However, in another study which used a standardized diagnostic interview, no association between a drug injection history and psychiatric diagnosis was found (McKinnon *et al.*, 1996). Behavioral factors may be more important determinants of drug injection among psychiatric patients than clinical features. In a group of chronically ill psychiatric patients without comorbid substance use disorders, rates of injection were not predicted by psychiatric diagnosis, chronicity, level of functioning, or psychiatric symptoms, but were predicted by a history of drug sniffing (Horwath, Cournos, McKinnon, Guido & Herman, 1996).

Lower AIDS knowledge scores have been associated with schizophrenia spectrum diagnoses and, in a separate study, with greater risk activity, although these associations were not found in other studies (McKinnon *et al.*, 1996). The role of specific aspects of psychiatric illness was examined in only one study which assessed the relative contributions of psychiatric symptoms and AIDS knowledge to unsafe behavior among people with serious mental illness. It found that better AIDS knowledge predicted only a greater likelihood of being sexually active but no other risk behavior, suggesting that sexually active patients may have more motivation than abstinent patients to attend to relevant HIV-related information (McKinnon et al., 1996).

Some situations unique to people with serious mental illness may increase the likelihood of exposure to HIV. Institutionalization, for example, may confer risk (Gounis, Conover & Roche, 1994). Recurrent hospitalization can interrupt long-term relationships, reinforcing the tendency to have unfamiliar partners. In addition, extended periods of hospitalization on same-sex units may foster same-sex activity which is particularly risky for men; in fact any sexual intercourse between patients may increase the risk of exposure to HIV because sex between patients often occurs in a relatively closed system where HIV is likely to be prevalent. Sexual intercourse between psychiatric inpatients, which tends to be underreported and has not been examined since the AIDS epidemic began, has been documented among less than one percent of patients during the prior year to two years (Akhtar Crocker, Docleu, Helfrich & Rheubau, 1977; Modestin, 1981). Among people with serious mental illness who live in the community, 10% met a sex partner in the past year at a mental health center (Kelly et al., 1992).

Institutional obstacles to condom acquisition are likely to impede patients' initiative to practice safer sex. Distribution of condoms to inpatients remains controversial. However, making condoms available to all patients, including inpatients who have off-ward privileges or who continue to engage in risk behaviors on the ward despite assertive attempts to intervene (Carmen & Brady, 1990), is an important and cost-effective primary prevention intervention. Many outpatient facilities don't have the resources or commitment to dispense enough condoms to their clients. This puts patients, who may encounter sexual and drug-use networks in urban treatment settings, at a disadvantage when they try to enact safer behaviors.

Other factors that increase risk: People with persistent or recurrent serious mental illness typically live in poor, urban neighborhoods with high concentrations of HIV and other sexually transmitted diseases and drug use, so the likelihood of coming into contact with an infected sex or drug-injection partner is increased (Kalichman, Sikkema, Kelly & Bulto, 1995). These and other environmental factors, including transient living circumstances and lack of privacy, may make AIDS prevention or the avoidance of risk behaviors a low priority or difficult to initiate for people with serious mental illness. Chronic debilitation and a concomitant lack of economic resources decrease the likelihood that people with serious mental illness who are sexually active can purchase condoms or that those who inject drugs will have their own works (Carmen & Brady, 1990).

Some risk situations are not unique to people with serious mental illness but may be experienced more frequently by them. Homelessness, alienation from supportive social relationships, or sexual victimization, may limit sexual opportunities to those that confer greater risk. Having unfamiliar sex partners, for example, decreases the likelihood of knowing their HIV status. Among psychiatric outpatients, five percent had sex in the past month with a partner they had known for less than one day (Kelly et al., 1992). Sex with prostitutes, who are at substantially increased risk of exposure to HIV, has been examined in a number of studies of people with serious mental illness. Buying sexual intercourse appears to be a fairly common practice among people in psychiatric treatment. Between 19% and 22% of inpatients and outpatients reported having sex, often unprotected, with a prostitute in the past year to five years (Carey et al., 1997). Despite the frequency of this behavior, intercourse with prostitutes may be less typical of the psychiatric population than the general population. One study found that 21% of psychiatric inpatients at a public general hospital reported having sex with a prostitute at some time in their lives, compared to 52% of a nonpsychiatric control group (McDermott et al., 1994). Another experience associated with HIV risk that is just beginning to be studied is sexual victimization, which increases the likelihood of unprotected intercourse (Herbert, 1995) and has been shown to be widespread among certain psychiatric inpatient groups (e.g., Danovsky, Brown, Kessel & Lipsitt, 1995). Among outpatients, 13% reported having been pressured and 14% having been coerced or forced into unwanted sex in the past year (Carey et al., 1997).

The risk of exposure to HIV is greater in certain locations where drug use occurs frequently. Urban neighborhoods, where many people with serious mental illness receive treatment, are often the site of high rates of drug injection. Shooting galleries, where needles and other works can be rented or traded, are common, and the likelihood of contact with HIV-infected injection equipment is high due to rapid turnover and poor cleaning practices (Marmor et al., 1987; Schoenbaum et al., 1989). Patronage of shooting galleries by people with serious mental illness remains an uninvestigated area of inquiry, and research is needed to identify factors that may encourage the sharing of injection equipment in this population. Factors thought most likely to affect psychiatric patients include limited availability of sterile equipment, economic motivation to share, and the role of sharing as part of friendship or bonding (Des Jarlais, Friedman, Strug & 1986; Murphy, 1987). The quality of street drugs also affects how people use them. If purer drugs are available they can be sniffed rather than injected to achieve the same degree of intoxication (French & Safford, 1989). Despite the potential protective effect of sniffing versus injection with regard to HIV exposure, sniffing may be a gateway to injecting because as addiction progresses, a larger dose of drug is needed to achieve the same degree of intoxication.

Prevention Interventions for People with Serious Mental Illness

Having learned that HIV infection is prevalent among adults in psychiatric treatment and that they engage in a wide variety of risky behaviors, several researchers developed and tested interventions for psychiatric patients designed to prevent the transmission and acquisition of HIV. Intensive, small-group programs that simultaneously target knowledge, attitudes, motivations, and cognitive and behavior skills have been tried and found to produce reductions in high-risk sexual behaviors (including some that are substance-related) among people with serious mental illness.

Effective elements from randomized outcome trials of these HIV risk reduction interventions (Kelly, 1997) include HIV risk education and skills training in sexual assertiveness, negotiation, problem-solving, use of condoms, and risk self-management (including identifying and monitoring personal risk "triggers" or situations in which risk behaviors are most likely to occur). Rates of unprotected intercourse following intervention declined by as much as 50% and the proportion of intercourse occasions protected by condoms increased from 18% to 53% (Kelly, 1997). Reductions also were reported in sexual contact with multiple partners and rates of unprotected sex (Kelly et al., 1997). The longest post-intervention behavior change was sustained for 18 months, although the magnitude of changes weakened considerably over that time (Susser, Miller et al., 1996) and among some patients began to drop off as early as two to three months after the intervention (Kalichman et al., 1995). This suggests that booster or maintenance sessions may be necessary to sustain safer behaviors. Effective interventions are intensive, running between six and 15 hours in duration to achieve reductions in high-risk behaviors, and being trained as an AIDS educator or advocate increased gains in safer behaviors by patients (Kelly, 1997).

HIV prevention programs that primarily dispense AIDS information have not been shown to influence risk behavior levels. From a practical standpoint, distributing booklets and pamphlets on HIV or lecturing patients about safer behavior is not by itself of much use (Cournos et al., 1997). Unless patients can personalize the risk, find the motivation to act more safely, and believe in their capacity to execute the skills needed to make appropriate changes, they are not likely to modify their behavior. Clinicians need to take an active approach, using the tested intervention models which are similar to psychosocial rehabilitation programs already in place for psychiatric patients (Kelly, 1997). This approach emphasizes repetition and booster sessions which are essential to facilitate and maintain change. Any treatment program for people with serious mental illness must provide AIDS prevention services if it wishes to consider itself comprehensive.

Most clinical programs can conduct a prevention intervention using the small-group format. Both professional and paraprofessional staff can lead these groups, provided that they have basic knowledge about HIV and that they are comfortable talking about sex and drug use. Most patients enjoy these groups when their sexual, cultural, religious, ethnic, and life-stage norms are respected (Cournos et al., 1997). This type of discussion, coupled with an engaging, interactive group format, will draw patients in and encourage active participation. Incentives such as food, small prizes, and transportation money also may be offered.

Mixed-gender groups may increase generalization from group exercises to real life situations for heterosexual patients and allow women to practice being assertive with men about having safer sex and avoiding unwanted sex. Single-gender groups can be useful for dealing with same-sex issues or for decreasing patients' anxiety about discussing sexual issues with the opposite sex. Sexually abstinent patients should also be encouraged to participate since they may not remain abstinent forever, may share what they have learned with friends and family members, or may validate for other patients the legitimate choice of an abstinent lifestyle.

Drug-related risk behaviors can be similarly addressed, with harm reduction as the ultimate goal of the intervention. Use of clean injection equipment and ways of minimizing sexual risk while high can be rehearsed in settings where institutional policies do not reinforce risky behaviors by making substance abuse treatment contingent on being totally drug-free (Cournos et al., 1997). If a program has a large enough number of HIV-positive patients, a separate support group can focus on the particular concerns of patients who are already HIV infected. However, these patients also can benefit from participating in regular prevention groups, and need not reveal their HIV status unless they wish to do so. Group leaders should leave time at the end of each session for participants to discuss personal issues privately and to address patients' needs by making appropriate referrals, including to HIV test sites.

TREATING HIV-INFECTED PEOPLE WITH SERIOUS MENTAL ILLNESS IN MENTAL HEALTH SETTINGS

Determining Who is HIV-Infected

The prevalence of HIV infection among people with serious mental illness makes identifying intimate behaviors known to increase the risk of transmission a critical public health endeavor and can be an important prevention intervention for individual patients. Unsafe behaviors can easily go undetected, especially when clinicians are reluctant to ask patients about them. Mental health care providers often play a pivotal role in helping patients access HIV testing, treatment, and prevention opportunities.

The first step in this process is to obtain a risk history, which should cover the frequency of sexual intercourse (vaginal, anal & oral); the number, gender, and known HIV risks of sex partners; whether the patient has traded sex (for money, drugs, a place to stay, cigarettes or other goods); past history and current symptoms of sexually transmitted diseases; use of condoms and other contraceptive methods; use of drugs, particularly those that are injected or sniffed; and sharing of needles, syringes, or other injection equipment. Rather than asking, "Have you ever...," asking "How often have you..." is more likely to elicit useful risk information without raising a patient's defenses by implying that the interviewer will judge such behaviors negatively or consider them unusual (McKinnon, 1996).

The point of the risk assessment is to elicit behaviorally specific information about patients' sexual behaviors and drug use. In spite of the sensitive nature of the subject matter, most patients, when asked in a direct and nonjudgmental way, are cooperative and forthcoming (Volavka et al., 1992). The ease the clinician demonstrates in discussing sex and drug use will set the anxiety level for the patient, and normalizing any patient discomfort can set a more relaxed tone. Key elements of effective risk behavior assessment (McKinnon, 1996) are sensitivity to differences in language (including sexual vocabulary), maintaining privacy and confidentiality, demonstrating cultural competence, and securing administrative support for the task. The assessment process is an important opportunity for patients to learn about HIV risk and prevention, and most patients can benefit from discussing sexual issues and relationships constructively with their mental health care providers (Sadow & Corman, 1983). Assessing risk behaviors regularly can open up a dialogue through which mental health care providers communicate their commitment to helping patients reduce their risk of acquiring or transmitting HIV infection.

Counseling HIV-Affected Psychiatric Patients

HIV antibody test counseling: Mental health care providers should offer to refer patients for HIV testing on a regular basis and whenever a patient asks for it, has current or past risk behaviors, is pregnant, has physical signs suggestive of HIV infection or AIDS, has psychiatric symptoms that suggest central nervous system (CNS) dysfunction, or has a positive PPD (Mantoux) test and resides in an area endemic for HIV (Oquendo & Tricarico, 1996). People with serious mental illness usually can undergo HIV counseling and antibody testing without distress or worsening of their psychiatric symptoms. Nevertheless, patients may require more than the single session of counseling and will need careful assessment of their capacity to consent to testing, and special issues may arise in the process of counseling them about their HIV status. While home HIV testing kits are now available for performing anonymous testing for HIV by mailing in a blood sample obtained with a lance, this approach is not encouraged with severely ill psychiatric patients (Cournos et al., 1997).

HIV test counselors must be knowledgeable about both HIV and the symptoms of mental illness and prepared to deal with some of the severe reactions that occasionally arise. Patients should undergo test counseling when their psychiatric condition permits, although HIV testing often can proceed when a patient is in the hospital for treatment of an acute episode. In fact, appropriate testing of inpatients has some advantages when the entire process can be completed before hospital discharge. In these cases, staff can ensure that patients receive post-test counseling and follow-up appointments, provide a buffer against the stress that HIV testing can precipitate, and address any worsening of the patient's psychiatric condition in the event of a distressing test result.

Many states have legal regulations for pre- and post-test counseling for HIV testing. These regulations serve as guidelines for confidentiality and the disclosure of HIV- or AIDS-related information, and set the stage for upholding humane and responsible individual and public health standards. Voluntary testing is the norm for people with serious mental illness so that those who are HIV positive can seek treatment and change their risk behaviors and yet be protected against discrimination. The capacity to consent to testing hinges on the ability to understand the information being conveyed and to draw reasonable conclusions from it, and people with serious mental illness are considered to have this capacity unless an assessment determines otherwise, in which case consent may be given by a person who is legally authorized to do so. Informed consent for HIV antibody testing should include an explanation of the test, its purpose, the meaning of the results, and the benefits of early diagnosis and medical intervention. In addition, explanation should be given of the voluntary nature of the test, the individual's right to withdraw consent at any time, the availability of anonymous testing, and confidentiality and the circumstances under which test results may be disclosed with or without the individual's agreement (Oquendo & Tricarico, 1996).

At pre-test, it is important to discuss AIDS and HIV-related illnesses, as well as possible discrimination that may occur if test results are revealed, and legal protections against discrimination. The patient's risk history should be obtained, which will require an open and explicit discussion of sexual behavior and substance use. This also provides an opportunity to correct any misconceptions regarding routes of transmission and what constitutes safer behavior. The patient's plans in the event of either a positive or negative test result should be elicited to determine appropriate timing for the antibody test and maximize the patients' readiness for the result. Many patients will do best when HIV test counseling is conducted at the mental health program by providers who have an existing relationship with the patient.

At post-test, results should be given with counseling, and where appropriate, additional referrals for counseling to facilitate coping with the emotional consequences of learning the positive, negative, or, on occasion, inconclusive result. Any test result, not just those that confirm the presence of HIV antibodies, may arouse anxiety, denial, suicidality, depression, assaultiveness or reappearance of psychiatric symptoms. The counselor should ask all patients to explain their understanding of the results, and correct any misconceptions. Counselors also should be prepared to help patients adapt to the uncertainties they face. For example, HIV-negative patients who have had risk behavior that is too recent for seroconversion to have occurred will need to be re-tested. Those with inconclusive results will also need help adjusting to the ambiguity of this finding and the possibility of repeated inconclusive results. For HIV-positive patients, assessing the immune system (viral load and CD4-cell count) should be stressed, available medical treatments described, and referrals to health care providers given. Support for obtaining adequate medical treatment may also be required. It is essential to discuss behavior changes needed to prevent transmission or contraction of HIV infection.

Partner notification: HIV-positive patients need to notify their at-risk sex and/or drug-injection partners. Patients may be able to notify partners independently or they may need assistance from clinicians. Clinicians can help reluctant patients to overcome their concerns about engaging in direct discussion with partners, and can offer to be present. This approach underscores the importance of counseling patients to help them understand how to protect sex and drug-injection partners and feel motivated to do so. Contact notification by physicians is not required in most states, but procedures as specified in state statutes may be allowed if a doctor determines that a patient will not do so and that the contact is at significant risk (Haimowitz, 1996). These statutes should be consulted. Patients should be aware of discrimination problems that can result from disclosure of positive HIV status. Some patients will need advice about when to withhold their HIV status from individuals (e.g., landlords, employers) who do not have a need to know.

Permanency planning: Psychiatric patients who test positive and have custody of small children will need assistance planning for their future care. The term permanency planning is now used to describe this process, which should include normalizing such planning so that it is seen as a necessary procedure for all parents, whether ill or not; ensuring that the designated caretaker(s) agrees to the plan; and completing the required legal documents and procedures to finalize it.

Supportive counseling or psychotherapy: The initial diagnosis of HIV infection may occur when a patient is asymptomatic, has advanced AIDS, or any time in between. Shock and disbelief may be followed by depression, anxiety, and fear (Bartlett, 1993) in adjusting to having contracted a terminal illness. Untreated depression and hopelessness are associated with continuing risk behavior and suicidal ideation (Liberman et al., 1986). Like serious mental illness, HIV and AIDS can be highly stigmatizing, possibly resulting in rejection, abandonment, and further social isolation (Empfield, 1996). A worsening of psychotic symptoms also may follow the initial HIV diagnosis. Under these circumstance, the most effective intervention is individual counseling and supportive therapy geared to both the current mental status of the patient and his or her knowledge and understanding of HIV infection (Broder, Merigan & Bolognesi, 1994). Psychiatric patients, like medical patients, are often noncompliant with their medication, which they may perceive as one of the few aspects of their lives they can control, so it is important to help patients see that following an HIV/AIDS medication regimen can be part of gaining such control (Empfield, 1996).

For HIV-infected psychiatric patients who are asymptomatic, supportive groups most effectively encourage behavioral change and promote ways to preserve physical health either in the community or within the psychiatric setting. Group intervention can prevent worsening of psychiatric symptoms and provide a sense of community that can decrease social isolation, reinforce safer peer norms, and encourage altruism which appeals to ego strengths and gives patients a sense of worth and accomplishment (Empfield, 1996).

Diagnosis and Management of HIV and AIDS

HIV-infected patients have an opportunity to accept what is now known as highly active antiretroviral treatment (HAART), a selected combination of antiretroviral agents that are used to maximally suppress viral replication and preserve immune function (Carpenter et al., 1997). Ideally HAART regimens should begin long before the patient is clinically ill because by that point the immune system is usually already severely damaged. Although a prolonged asymptomatic period usually follows initial infection, lasting nine to 10 years on average, during this time viral replication is nonetheless active and ongoing and the immune system is weakening. The time interval from infection to symptom onset is quite variable and probably depends on route of infection, general health, and immune status prior to HIV infection, among other factors. The purpose of HAART is to prevent irreversible immune deficits (Carpenter et al., 1997). Disease progression can be monitored by repeated measures of viral load (the amount of circulating virus in the blood) and CD4+ T-lymphocyte counts (the primary white blood cell involved in the body's immune system response to HIV). The higher the viral load and the lower the

CD4-cell count, the worse the outlook is for the patient. These biological markers are followed for the purpose of adjusting the HAART regimen and beginning prophylactic medications in a timely way to prevent HIV-related opportunistic infections. Pregnant women who know they are HIV positive can take antiretroviral treatment during pregnancy, delivery, and/or the post-partum period. This strategy dramatically reduces the chances of a woman passing HIV infection on to her baby.

The onset of physical signs or symptoms of illness such as weight loss or lymphadenopathy, after a long period of relatively healthy functioning, may precipitate psychiatric symptoms. Progression from minor symptoms to major illness, such as opportunistic infection or neoplasm, is also a significant event. HIV infection presents a spectrum of medical and neuropsychiatric sequelae which can pose diagnostic and treatment quandaries to mental health clinicians. In patients with severe and chronic psychiatric illness, some of the early, subtle neuropsychiatric symptoms may be difficult to differentiate from pre-existing symptoms of their psychiatric illness. Both HIV and the many opportunistic infections and neoplasms that follow immunosuppression also can affect the CNS, resulting in mood disorders, psychosis, cognitive disorders, HIV-related dementia, delirium, and other neurological or systemic abnormalities. In addition, prescribed and recreational psychoactive substance use may create neuropsychiatric complications and must be considered in the differential diagnosis of patients who present such symptoms (McDaniel, Purcell & Farber, 1997).

Central Nervous System Complications

The AIDS virus is neurotropic (O'Brien, 1994), that is, it crosses the blood-brain barrier and directly affects the brain. HIV enters the CNS soon after infection (Resnick, Berger, Shapshak & Tourtellotte, 1988) but is rarely diagnosed at this time. The CNS manifestation of acute HIV infection is headache with or without meningeal signs. Over time, clinical manifestations of CNS infection range from subtle neurocognitive impairment to frank dementia. Many complicating medical illnesses that patients develop later in the course of disease progression when they become immunocompromised involve the brain and can mimic psychiatric conditions. Table 7.1 summarizes the most common CNS manifestations of HIV infection.

HIV infection also causes systemic immunosuppression which results in a variety of opportunistic infections that are unusual in the absence of HIV and tend to occur late in the course of illness, when immune function is waning and CD4+ cell counts fall to very low levels. The identification of the underlying cause of neuropsychiatric disturbance in an HIV-infected person is very important because some opportunistic infections are responsive to treatment, which can restore

Table 7.1. Common Central Nervous System Manifestations of HIV Infection.

Direct effects of HIV	headache
	aseptic meningitis
	HIV-associated minor cognitive-motor disorder (MCMD)
	HIV-associated dementia (HAD)
	neuropsychiatric sequelae not meeting criteria for MCMD or HAD
Opportunistic infections	*viral*
	cytomegalovirus (CMV) encephalitis
	varicella-zoster encephalitis
	herpes simplex encephalitic
	progressive multifocal leukoencephalopathy (PML)
	non-viral
	cerebral toxoplasmosis
	cryptococcal meningitis
Opportunistic neoplasms	primary CNS lymphoma (EBV-related)
	secondary CNS lymphoma
	metastatic Kaposi's sarcoma
Metabolic disorders	hypoxic encephalopathy
	encephalopathy secondary to sepsis
HIV-related medication-induced disorders	cognitive disorders (e.g., confusion, encephalopathy)
	mood disorders (depression, mania)
	perceptual disorders (e.g., hallucinations)
	systemic disorders (e.g., agitation, fatigue, insomnia)

the patient to his or her previous state of functioning (Horwath, 1996). A number of non-viral opportunistic infections may mimic neuropsychiatric syndromes ranging from mood disorders to cognitive impairment and delirium. Cerebral toxoplasmosis, an intracellular protozoan (parasitic) infection, is the most common CNS opportunistic infection in people with AIDS, occurring in five percent to 20% of late-stage AIDS patients (Horwath, 1996) and usually presenting with ring-enhancing lesions clearly distinguishable on computerized tomography scan or magnetic resonance imaging (American Psychiatric Association [APA], 1996). Treatment is generally effective, especially if begun early, but requires lifelong prophylactic medication following resolution of the initial infection.

Cryptococcossis is the most common CNS fungal infection in AIDS, occurring in five percent to 15% of AIDS patients (Horwath, 1996) and usually producing a classic meningitis. It has been linked to numerous neuropsychiatric complications including mania (McDaniel *et al.*, 1997). Cryptococcal meningitis is generally treatable with antifungal medications, and like toxoplasmosis, requires lifelong prophylactic treatment after initial infection or when the level of immunosuppression reaches a high risk point (McDaniel *et al.*, 1997). Other non-viral infections include brain involvement of tuberculosis or atypical mycobacterium (MAI), CNS candida infections, and neurosyphilis.

The most common viral opportunistic infections in HIV disease belong to the herpes virus family. These viruses, cytomegalovirus (CMV), varicella-zoster virus (VZ), and herpes simplex virus (HSV), can produce severe, life-threatening brain infections. Of these, CMV encephalitis is the most common infection, but may be the most under-recognized due to difficulties in diagnosis and because the presentation is frequently confused with HIV-associated dementia (McDaniel *et al.*, 1997). CMV encephalitis also remains difficult to treat as the role of current antiviral agents remains undefined (McDaniel *et al.*, 1997). VZ and HSV infections are extremely serious in immunocompromised individuals, but are more readily diagnosable and usually treatable. Progressive multifocal leukoencephalopathy (PML) is a rare but serious demyelinating complication caused by reactivation of a latent papovavirus (the JC virus). PML presents with focal neurological deficits (aphasia, ataxia & hemiparesis) and cognitive impairment that progresses to death over weeks or a few months (McDaniel *et al.*, 1997); current treatments have not proven effective for this condition (APA, 1996).

Opportunistic neoplasms or tumors present a serious challenge to immunocompromised patients and remain an important consideration in the diagnosis of new onset neuropsychiatric complications. Primary CNS lymphoma, a rare tumor prior to the emergence of AIDS, is a more commonly seen CNS cancer in persons with AIDS, second only to toxoplasmosis as a cause of intracranial mass lesions (APA, 1996). Typical presentation involves slow and progressive neurological deterioration accompanied by such mental status changes as confusion, lethargy, and memory loss, leading to death within months (McDaniel *et al.*, 1997). Treatment is generally palliative and consists of radiation, as well as chemotherapy in select cases. Other malignancies in the brain include secondary CNS lymphoma that has metastasized from other body regions (e.g., the lung or gastrointestinal tract), and metastatic Kaposi's sarcoma (a tumor which generally manifests on the skin or mouth). These secondary neoplasms are less common than primary CNS lymphoma.

Encephalopathies linked to systemic or metabolic conditions occur frequently in patients with AIDS, particularly when opportunistic pulmonary infections cause hypoxia or when multiorgan failure develops (McDaniel *et al.*, 1997). This is often seen in patients with *Pneumocystis carinii*. Many medical complications in AIDS, including fever, dehydration, anemia, and blood infections can manifest with psychiatric symptoms. In such cases, the primary treatment is aggressive management of the underlying medical condition as well as provision of a sensitive, supportive environment to these patients who may be confused or anxious (McDaniel *et al.*, 1997).

Diagnostic criteria: HIV-related neuropsychiatric diagnoses are diagnoses of exclusion made after all other etiologies have been ruled out, and should involve a neurological evaluation. Cognitive disorders in HIV infection can be divided into three categories. Minor cognitive-motor disorder (MCMD) is a mild syndrome of motor and/or cognitive dysfunction with minimal impairment in functioning (McDaniel *et al.*, 1997). The diagnosis can be made if any two of the following are present: Impaired attention or concentration, mental slowing, impaired memory, slowed movements, impaired coordination, or personality change, irritability, or lability. MCMD does not progress necessarily to HIV-associated dementia (HAD), a more severe disorder (Masliah, Achim, DeTeresa & Wiley, 1996). Criteria for HAD include acquired cognitive abnormality in two or more cognitive domains causing functional impairment; acquired abnormality in motor performance or decline in motivation or emotional control; no clouding of consciousness (delirium); and no confounding etiology, including active CNS opportunistic infection, psychiatric disorder, or active substance abuse. HAD is relatively common, particularly in more advanced stages of HIV infection (McDaniel *et al.*, 1997). In adults, dementia rarely occurs before the onset of other AIDS-defining illnesses. The exact pathophysiology of HAD remains unclear. Patients may also have neuropsychiatric impairments that do not meet criteria for MCMD or HAD.

Combining Medical and Psychiatric Treatments

HIV-related psychopharmacological interventions for people with pre-existing mental illness follow similar guidelines for patients with new-onset psychosis secondary to HIV infection. Traditional neuroleptic agents have been found to produce modest but significant reductions in psychotic symptoms with careful dosing for potential side effects (generally lower doses are used with HIV-infected patients than with non-infected patients) (Sewell *et al.*, 1994; Fernandez & Levy, 1993). People with preexisting psychiatric conditions may develop new or increased side effects on medications they were previously able to tolerate (Horwath, 1996). Severe extrapyramidal side effects (EPS) often follow administration of standard highpotency neuroleptics (American Psychiatric Association HIV/AIDS Practice Guideline, in preparation).

Atypical antipsychotic agents such as risperidone and olanzapine may be particularly helpful in treating these individuals due to favorable side effect and dosage profiles (Apter, 1996).

HIV medication options: A large number of medications are prescribed to people with HIV infection, including antibacterial, antifungal, antineoplastic, antiretroviral and other antiviral agents (Horwath, 1996), particularly in later stages of HIV disease when numerous complications require active treatment.

To treat HAD, two pharmacological approaches to treatment have been used. First, antiretroviral drugs such as zidovudine (AZT) are given to treat the primary viral infection to improve cognitive functioning by directly affecting HIV, particularly within the CNS. There are limited data that other antiretroviral agents (e.g. didanosine, zalcitabine) may be of some benefit in treating HAD (Yarchoan *et al.*, 1990), but systematic investigations of the newest class of antiretrovirals (protease inhibitors) are lacking. The second line of pharmacological treatment utilizes psychostimulants. This treatment targets the symptoms of HAD, especially those involving impairment in attention and concentration, particularly when accompanied by apathy or depressed mood. Psychostimulants such as methylphenidate have been studied extensively in HIV-positive patients and have been found to be well tolerated and to lead to a decrease in cognitive and depressive symptoms associated with dementia (Fernandez, Levy & Ruiz, 1994). For patients with HAD who also develop psychotic features, a condition for which psychostimulants are contraindicated, low doses of neuroleptic medications may be efficacious in managing symptoms (APA, 1996). There are many other investigational drugs currently under study for HAD, and it is important to keep track of the latest advances when treating patients with this condition.

Neuropsychiatric side effects of AIDS treatments: Neuropsychiatric side effects of AIDS medications can range from mild symptoms of insomnia or irritability to severe symptoms of depression, mania, or psychosis (McDaniel *et al.*, 1997). Any attempt to diagnose drug-induced neuropsychiatric syndromes requires an appreciation of both the therapeutic use and potential side effects of these medications. Some of these are shown in Table 7.1, but new antiretroviral agents are being developed at a rapid pace and existing medications to treat HIV-related infections and neoplasms are too numerous to describe fully.

Antipsychotic-Antiviral Drug Interactions

Triple-drug therapy to reduce viral load is promising but the protease inhibitors approved by the Food and Drug Administration all must be carefully administered in conjunction with psychotropic agents and evaluated on a case-by-case basis. For a detailed description of indications for the use of these medications, we refer you to the curriculum on HIV-related neuropsychiatric complications and treatments of the American Psychiatric Association (1996). Because protease inhibitors are relatively new medications, a literature is only now evolving to guide clinicians' prescribing practices. Ritonavir, for example, is a potent inhibitor of cytochrome p450 (3A4) and thus when co-administered with medications that are highly metabolized by cytochrome p450, such as tricyclic antidepressants or the anxiolytics alprazolam, clonazepam, and kiazapam, its dosage must be reduced or the agent discontinued. Drug-drug interactions will require adjustments for many other agents.

IN CONCLUSION

In this chapter we presented a range of issues that mental health care providers must address with their patients in the age of AIDS. We hope that the epidemiological evidence will increase providers' awareness of HIV infection and their confidence that they can help their patients determine their personal risk of acquiring or transmitting the AIDS virus. Providers can use the prevention strategies we described to help their uninfected patients remain HIV-negative and keep their HIV-positive patients healthy and emotionally well-functioning. We also described the impact of HIV on psychiatric illness and provided management and medication guidelines which we hope will result in integrated care for people with serious mental illness affected by HIV and AIDS.

REFERENCES

Akhtar, S., Crocker, E., Docleu, N., Helfrich, J. & Rheubau, W.J. (1977). Overt sexual behavior among psychiatric inpatients. *Diseases of the Nervous System* 38:359–361.

Akhtar, S. & Thomson, J.A. (1980). Schizophrenia and sexuality: A review and a report of twelve unusual cases – part II. *Journal of Clinical Psychiatry* 41:166–174.

American Psychiatric Association (1996). *HIV-related Neuropsychiatric Complications and Treatments: HIV/AIDS Training Curriculum.* Washington, DC.

American Psychiatric Association (in preparation). HIV/AIDS Practice Guideline.

Apter, J.T. (1996). A new generation of antipsychotics emerges. *Primary Psychiatry* 3:22–23.

Auerbach, J.D., Wypijewska, C. & Brodie, H.K.H. (Eds.) (1994). *AIDS and Behavior: An Integrated Approach.* Washington, DC: National Academy Press.

Bartlett, J.G. (1993). *The Guide to Living with HIV Infection: Developed at the Johns Hopkins AIDS Clinic,* rev. ed. Baltimore: Johns Hopkins University Press.

Broder, S., Merigan, T.C. & Bolognesi, D. (Eds.) (1994). *Textbook of AIDS Medicine.* Baltimore: Williams & Wilkins.

Carey, M.P., Carey, K.B. & Kalichman, S.C. (1997). Risk for Human Immunodeficiency Virus (HIV) infection among persons with severe mental illnesses. *Clinical Psychology Review* 17:271–291.

Carmen, E. & Brady, S.M. (1990). AIDS risk and prevention for the chronic mentally ill. *Hospital and Community Psychiatry* 41:652–657.

Carpenter, C.C., Fischl, M.A., Hammer, S.M., Hirsch, M.S., Jacobsen, D.M., Katzenstein, D.A., Montaner, J.S., Richman, D.D., Saag, M.S., Schooley, R.T., Thompson, M.A., Vella, S., Yeni, P.G. & Volberding, P.A. (1997). Antiretroviral therapy for HIV infection in 1997. Updated recommendations of the International AIDS Society-USA panel. *Journal of the American Medical Association* 277:1962–1969.

Conant, M.A. (1984). Speculations on the viral etiology of acquired immune deficiency syndrome and Kaposi's sarcoma. *Journal of Investigative Dermatology* 83:57s–62s.

Cournos, F., Empfield, M., Horwath, E., McKinnon, K., Meyer, I., Schrage, H., Currie, C. & Agosin, B. (1991). HIV seroprevalence among patients admitted to two psychiatric hospitals. *American Journal of Psychiatry* 148: 1225–1230.

Cournos, F., Guido, J.R., Coomaraswamy, S., Meyer-Bahlburg, H.F.L., Sugden, R. & Horwath, E. (1994). Sexual activity and risk of HIV infection among patients with schizophrenia. *American Journal of Psychiatry* 151:228–232.

Cournos, F., Herman, R., Kaplan, M. & McKinnon, K. (1997). AIDS prevention for people with severe mental illness. *Journal of Practical Psychiatry and Behavioral Health* 3:285–292.

Cournos, F. & McKinnon, K. (1997). HIV seroprevalence among people with severe mental illness in the United States: A critical review. *Clinical Psychology Review* 17:259–269.

Cournos, F., McKinnon, K., Meyer-Bahlburg, H.F.L., Guido, J.R. & Meyer, I. (1993). HIV risk activity among persons with severe mental illness: Preliminary findings. *Hospital and Community Psychiatry* 44:1104–1106.

Danovsky, M., Brown, L., Kessel, S. & Lipsitt, L. (1995). Psychiatrically hospitalized adolescents: Sexual-abuse as a co-factor in HIV risk. In Abstracts (FE1-187), *HIV Infection in Women: Setting a New Agenda*. Washington, DC: Philadelphia Sciences Group.

Des Jarlais, D.C., Friedman, S.R. & Strug, D. (1986). AIDS and needle sharing within the intravenous drug use subculture. In Feldman, D. and Johnson, T. (Eds.), *The Social Dimensions of AIDS: Methods and Theory*. New York: Praeger.

Empfield, M. (1996). Working with HIV-infected people. In Cournos, F. and Bakalar, N.(Eds.), *AIDS and People with Severe Mental Illness: A Handbook for Mental Health Professionals*. New Haven: Yale University Press.

Empfield, M., Cournos, F., Meyer, I., McKinnon, K., Horwath, E., Silver, M., Shrage, H. & Herman, R. (1993). HIV seroprevalence among homeless patients admitted to a psychiatric inpatient unit. *American Journal of Psychiatry* 150:47–52.

Fernandez, F. & Levy, J.K. (1993). The use of molindone in the treatment of psychotic and delirious patients infected with the human immunodeficiency virus: Case reports. *General Hospital Psychiatry* 15:31–35.

Fernandez, F., Levy, J.K. & Ruiz, P. (1994). The use of methylphenidate in HIV patients: A clinical perspective. In Grant, I. and Martin, A. (Eds.), *Neuropsychology of HIV Infection*. New York: Oxford University Press.

French, J.F. & Safford, J. (1989). AIDS and intranasal heroin (letter). *Lancet* 1: 1082.

Gewirtz, G.R., Horwath, E., Cournos, F. & Empfield, M. (1988). Patients at risk for HIV (letter). *Hospital and Community Psychiatry* 39:1311–1312.

Gounis, K., Conover, S. & Roche, B. (1994). Homelessness in New York City: The institutional determinants of HIV risk behaviors. In Abstracts (S5.2), *2nd International Conference on AIDS' Impact: Biopsychosocial Aspects of HIV Infection.* Brighton, England.

Haimowitz, S. (1996). An overview of legal issues. In Cournos, F. and Bakalar, N. (Eds.), *AIDS and People with Severe Mental Illness: A Handbook for Mental Health Professionals.* New Haven: Yale University Press.

Hanson, M., Kramer, T.H., Gross, W., Quintana, J., Li, P. & Asher, R. (1992). AIDS awareness and risk behaviors among dually disordered adults. *AIDS Education and Prevention* 4:41–51.

Hardy, A.M. (1990). National health interview survey data on adult knowledge AIDS in the United States. *Public Health Report* 105:629–634.

Herbert, B. (1995). Woman battering and HIV infection. In Abstracts (TP500), *HIV Infection in Women: Setting a New Agenda.* Washington, DC: Philadelphia Sciences Group.

Horwath, E. (1996). Psychiatric and neuropsychiatric manifestations. In Cournos, F. and Bakalar, N. (Eds.), *AIDS and People with Severe Mental Illness: A Handbook for Mental Health Professionals.* New Haven: Yale University Press.

Horwath, E., Cournos, F., McKinnon, K., Guido, J.R. & Herman, R. (1996). Illicit-drug injection among psychiatric patients without a primary substance use disorder. *Psychiatric Services* 47:181–185.

Kalichman, S.C., Kelly, J.A., Johnson, J.R. & Bulto, M. (1994). Factors associated with risk for HIV infection among chronic mentally ill adults. *American Journal of Psychiatry* 151:221–227.

Kalichman, S.C., Sikkema, K.J., Kelly, J.A. & Bulto, M. (1995). Use of a brief behavioral skills intervention to prevent HIV infection among chronic mentally ill adults. *Psychiatric Services* 46:275–280.

Kelly, J.A. (1997). HIV risk reduction interventions for persons with severe mental illness. *Clinical Psychology Review* 17:293–309.

Kelly, J.A., Murphy, D.A., Bahr, G.R., Brasfield, T.L., Davis, D.R., Hauth, A.C., Morgan, M.G., Stevenson, L.Y. & Eilers, M.K. (1992). AIDS/HIV risk behavior among the chronic mentally ill. *American Journal of Psychiatry* 149:886–889.

Kim, A., Galanter, M., Castaneda, R., Lifshutz, H. & Franco, H. (1992). Crack cocaine use and sexual behavior among psychiatric inpatients. *American Journal of Drug and Alcohol Abuse* 18:235–246.

Klaf, F.S. (1961). Female homosexuality and paranoid schizophrenia: A survey of 75 cases and controls. *Archives of General Psychiatry* 4:84–86.

Klaf, F.S. & Davis, C.A. (1960). Homosexuality and paranoid schizophrenia: A survey of 105 cases and controls. *American Journal of Psychiatry* 116:1070–1075.

Laumann, E.O., Gagnon, J.H., Michael, R.T. & Michaels, S. (1994). *The Social Organization of Sexuality.* Chicago, IL: University of Chicago Press.

Lee, H.K., Travin, S. & Bluestone, H. (1992). HIV-1 in inpatients. *Hospital and Community Psychiatry* 43:181–182.

Leigh, C.B. (1990). The relationship of substance use during sex to high-risk behavior. *Journal of Sex Research* 27:199–213.

Liberman, R.P., Mueser, K.T., Wallace, C.J., Jacobs, H.E., Eckman, T. & Massell, H.K. (1986). Training skills in the psychiatrically disabled: Learning coping and competence. *Schizophrenia Bulletin* 12:631–647.

Lukianowicz, N. (1963). Sexual drive and its gratification in schizophrenia. *International Journal of Social Psychiatry* 9:250–258.

Lukoff, D., Gioia-Hasiok, D., Sullivan, G., Golden, J.S. & Neuchterlein, K.H. (1986). Sex education and rehabilitation with schizophrenic male outpatients. *Schizophrenia Bulletin* 12:669–677.

Lyketsos, G.C., Sakka, P. & Mailis, A. (1983). The sexual adjustment of chronic schizophrenics: A preliminary study. *British Journal of Psychiatry* 143:376–382.

Marmor, M., Des Jarlais, D.C., Cohen, H., Friedman, S.R., Beatrice, S.T., Dubin, N., el-Sadr, W., Mildvan, D., Yancovitz, S., Mathur, U. & Holzman, R. (1987). Risk factors for infection with human immunodeficiency virus among intravenous drug abusers in New York City. *AIDS* 1:39–44.

Masliah, G., Achim, C.L., DeTeresa, R. & Wiley, C.A. (1996). The patterns of neurodegeneration in HIV encephalitis. *Journal of NeuroAIDS* 1:161–173.

McDaniel, J.S., Purcell, D.W. & Farber, E.W. (1997). Severe mental illness and HIV-related medical and neuropsychiatric sequelae. *Clinical Psychology Review* 17:311–325.

McDermott, B.E., Sautter, F.J., Winstead, D.K. & Quirk, T. (1994). Diagnosis, health beliefs,and risk of HIV infection in psychiatric patients. *Hospital and Community Psychiatry* 45:580–585.

McKeganey, N., Barnard, M. & Watson, H. (1989). HIV-related risk behavior among a non-clinic sample of injecting drug users. *British Journal of Addiction* 84:1481–1490.

McKinnon, K. (1996). Sexual and drug-use risk behavior. In Cournos F. and Bakalar N. (Eds.), *AIDS and People with Severe Mental Illness: A Handbook for Mental Health Professionals*. New Haven: Yale University Press.

McKinnon, K., Cournos, F., Sugden, R., Guido, J.R. & Herman, R. (1996). The relative contributions of psychiatric symptoms and AIDS knowledge to HIV risk behaviors among people with severe mental illness. *Journal of Clinical Psychiatry* 57:506–513.

Menon, A.S. & Pomerantz, S. (1997). Substance use during sex and unsafe sexual behaviors among acute psychiatric inpatients. *Psychiatric Services* 48:1070–1072.

Metsch, L. (1995). Health care utilization among HIV+ and HIV- women who are injection drug users. In Abstracts (WB365), *HIV Infection in Women: Setting a New Agenda*. Washington, DC: Philadelphia Sciences Group.

Meyer, I., Cournos, F., Empfield, M., Schrage, H., Silver, M., Rubin, M. & Weinstock, A. (1993). HIV seroprevalence and clinical characteristics of the mentally ill homeless. *Journal of Social Distress and the Homeless* 2: 103–116.

Meyer, I., McKinnon, K., Cournos, F., Empfield, M., Bavli, S., Engel, D. & Weinstock, A. (1993). HIV seroprevalence among long-stay psychiatric inpatients. *Hospital and Community Psychiatry* 44:282–284.

Modestin, J. (1981). Patterns of overt sexual interaction among acute psychiatric inpatients. *Acta Psychiatrica Scandanavia* 64:446–459.

Morningstar, P. & Chitwood, D. (1987). How women and men get cocaine: Sex-role stereotypes and acquisition patterns. *Journal of Psychoactive Drugs,* 19:135–142.

Murphy, S. (1987). Intravenous drug use and AIDS: Notes on the social economy of needle sharing. *Contemporary Drug Problems* 14:373–410.

O'Brien, W.A. (1994). Genetic and biologic basis of HIV-1 neurotropism. In Price, R.W. & Perry, S.W. (Eds.), *HIV, AIDS and The Brain*. New York: Raven Press, Ltd.

Oquendo, M. & Tricarico, P. (1996). Pre- and post-HIV test counseling. In Cournos F. and Bakalar N. (Eds.), *AIDS and People with Severe Mental Illness: A Handbook for Mental Health Professionals*. New Haven: Yale University Press.

Resnick, L., Berger, J.R., Shapshak, P. & Tourtellotte, W.W. (1988). Early penetration of the blood brain barrier by HTLV-III/LAV. *Neurology* 38: 9–15.

Sacks, M.H., Dermatis, H., Looser-Ott, S. & Perry, S. (1992). Seroprevalence of HIV and risk factors for AIDS in psychiatric inpatients. *Hospital and Community Psychiatry* 43:736–737.

Sacks, M.H., Perry, S., Graver, R., Shindledecker, R. & Hall, S. (1990). Self-reported HIV- related risk behaviors in acute psychiatric inpatients: A pilot study. *Hospital and Community Psychiatry* 41:1253–1255.

Sadow, D. & Corman, A.G. (1983). Teaching a human sexuality course to psychiatric patients: The process, pitfalls, and rewards. *Sexuality and Disability* 6:47–53.

Schoenbaum, E.E., Hartel, D., Selwyn, P.A., Klein, R.S., Davenny, K., Rogers, M., Feiner, C. & Friedland, G. (1989). Risk factors for human immunodeficiency virus infection in intravenous drug users. *New England Journal of Medicine* 321:874–879.

Schwartz-Watts, D., Montgomery, L.D. & Morgan, W. (1995). Seroprevalence of human immunodeficiency virus among inpatient pretrial detainees. *Bulletin of the American Academy of Psychiatry and the Law* 23: 285–288.

Sewell, D.D., Jeste, D.V., McAdams, L.A., Bailey, A., Harris, M.J., Atkinson, J.H., Chandler, J.L., McCutchan, J.A. & Grant, I. (1994). Neuroleptic treatment of HIV-associated psychosis. *Neuropsychopharmacology* 10:223–229.

Siegel, K. & Gibson, W. (1988). Barriers to the modification of sexual behavior among heterosexuals at risk for acquired immunodeficiency syndrome. *New York State Journal of Medicine* 88:66–70.

Silberstein, C., Galanter, M., Marmor, M., Lifshutz, H. & Krasinski, K. (1994). HIV-1 among inner city dually diagnosed inpatients. *American Journal of Drug and Alcohol Abuse* 20:101–131.

Stall, R., McKusick, L. & Wiley, J. (1986). Alcohol and drug use during sexual activity: Compliance with safe sex for AIDS. *Health Education Quarterly*, 13:359–371.

Steele, F.R. (1994). A moving target: CDC still trying to estimate HIV-1 prevalence. *Journal of NIH Research* 6:25–26.

Stevenson, L.Y., Murphy, D.A., Kelly, J.A., Fernandez, M.I., Miller, J.G. & Somlai, A.M. (1993). Risk characteristics for HIV infection among urban chronic mentally ill adults. In Abstracts (PO-C11-2857), *9th International Conference on AIDS*. Berlin, Germany.

Stewart, D.L., Zuckerman, C.J. & Ingle, J.M. (1994). HIV seroprevalence in a chronically mentally ill population. *Journal of the National Medical Association* 86:519–523.

Susser, E., Betne, P., Valencia, E., Goldfinger, S.M. & Lehman, A.F. (1997). Injection drug use among homeless adults with severe mental illness. *American Journal of Public Health* 87:854–856.

Susser, E., Colson, P., Jandorf, L., Berkman, A., Lavelle, J., Fennig, S., Waniek, C. & Bromet, E. (1997). HIV infection among young adults with psychotic disorders. *American Journal of Psychiatry* 154:864–866.

Susser, E., Miller, M., Valencia, E., Colson, P., Roche, B. & Conover, S. (1996). Injection drug use and risk of HIV transmission among homeless men with mental illness. *American Journal of Psychiatry* 153:794–798.

Susser, E., Valencia, E. & Conover, S. (1993). Prevalence of HIV infection among psychiatric patients in a New York City men's shelter. *American Journal of Public Health* 83:568–570.

van Ameijden, E.J.C., van den Hoek, J.A.R., Jartgers, C. & Coutinho, R.A. (1994). Risk factors for the transition from noninjection to injection drug use and accompanying AIDS risk behavior in a cohort of drug users. *American Journal of Epidemiology* 139:1153–1163.

Verhulst, J. & Schneidman, B. (1981). Schizophrenia and sexual functioning. *Hospital and Community Psychiatry* 32:259–262.

Volavka, J., Convit, A., Czobar, P., Douyon, R., O'Donnell, J. & Ventura, F. (1991). HIV seroprevalence and risk behaviors in psychiatric inpatients. *Psychiatry Research* 39:109–114.

Volavka, J., Convit, A., O'Donnell, J., Douyon, R., Evangelista, C. & Czobor, P. (1992). Assessment of risk behaviors for HIV infection among psychiatric inpatients. *Hospital and Community Psychiatry* 43:482–85.

Wortley, P.M. & Fleming, P.L. (1997). AIDS in women in the United States: Recent trends. *Journal of the American Medical Association* 278:911–916.

Yarchoan, R., Pluda, J.M., Thomas, R.V., Mitsuya, H., Brouwers, P., Wyvill, K.M., Hartman, N., Johns, D.G. & Broder, S. (1990). Long-term toxicity/activity profile of 1-2-dideooxyinosiine in AIDS or AIDS related complex. *Lancet* 336:526–529.

8

Sexual Trauma in Women with Severe and Persistent Mental Illness

STANLEY D. ROSENBERG, LISA
A. GOODMAN, KIM THOMPSON and
KIM T. MUESER

INTRODUCTION

The lack of adequate research data, combined with numerous biases and mythologies held by both the public and by professionals, has obscured our understanding of sexuality in the lives of people with severe and persistent mental illnesses (SPMI). This chapter will attempt to shed light on a particular area of past ignorance: the impact of sexual trauma and violent victimization on the lives of women with SPMI. Sexual abuse has a very high prevalence in this group, and is associated with changes in sexual behavior, psychopathology and other risky and self-harming behaviors.

Over the last decade, the general issue of violence against women, including sexual abuse, has increasingly become a focus of research and clinical interest. Although many clinicians have become sensitized to this issue, the research literature on sexual abuse and its correlates in women with SPMI has been scarce and rather fragmentary. Only in the last several years has a better articulated picture of the relationship between these complex issues begun to emerge. The available findings suggest that experiences of past and ongoing sexual assault and coercion are ubiquitous in many sectors of this vulnerable population, and their effects severe and far reaching. This may be especially the case in women with a so called "dual diagnosis": a severe mental illness combined with substance use disorder.

More than a dozen published studies provide consistent evidence of the elevated prevalence, and clinical significance, of sexual abuse experiences in women with SPMI (for a review, see Goodman, Rosenberg, Mueser & Drake, 1997b). In the populations of SPMI women studied to date, sexuality has been commonly linked with experiences of exploitation, coercion and violence. Multiple, rather than single traumas, are frequent, and sexual abuse has tended to occur both in these women's early development and in their ongoing experiences in the community. In the most vulnerable sub-populations, such as inner-city women with dual disorders (e.g., schizophrenia and crack cocaine addiction), sexual violence is so common as to be a normative experience. Moreover, when sex trading for food, shelter and other necessities becomes common because of psychiatric and/or substance abuse morbidity, the line between coerced and uncoerced sex becomes rather blurred. In addition, the mutual influences of basic psychopathology, sexual trauma, and substance use disorders are yet to be delineated. For example, chronic psychoses put women at risk for poverty and homelessness which are, in turn, risk factors for sexual assault and other forms of violent victimization. Sexual assault, on the other hand, increases risk for substance use disorder and depression, which may exacerbate the course of a pre-existing psychiatric disorder.

While exposure to abuse has been shown to correlate with multiple problems in general female populations, much less is known about the sequelae of childhood or adult sexual abuse in the SPMI population. It is of considerable clinical significance to conceptualize the relationships between sexual abuse, treatment response and course of illness in women with SPMI. Such a model might pave the way to the development of mental health and substance abuse treatment approaches which are more attuned to the special needs of women dealing with this array of problems. It is also necessary for the development of interventions designed to ameliorate the effects of sexual abuse in women with SPMI, thereby improving the overall quality of their lives.

This chapter begins by defining some key terms, and then reviewing research on the prevalence of sexual abuse both in general and in clinical populations of women with SPMI. Next, we discuss some of the common correlates of sexual abuse which have been reported in peer-reviewed studies. These include revictimization, post-traumatic stress disorder (PTSD), substance use disorders, homelessness, and HIV-related risky sexual behavior. We also present several hypotheses that help explain the links between these symptoms and sexual abuse trauma. Finally, we discuss the clinical implications of these findings.

Definitions of Child and Adult Sexual Abuse

Sexual abuse has been defined generally as sexual assault experiences sustained during childhood and/or adulthood and specifically as the forcible touching of breasts or genitals, forcible intercourse, and being forced to stimulate a perpetrator's genitalia, including anal, oral, or vaginal sex (Briere, 1984). Childhood sexual abuse has been defined in various studies as abuse taking place before the age of 16 or 18, and adult sexual abuse has been defined as abuse taking place after the age of 16 or 18 (Goodman *et al.*, 1997). In addition, most investigators define any sexual contact between a child and a person five years or more older as abusive.

Prevalence

It is difficult to obtain accurate estimates of the prevalence rates of the sexual abuse of women in the United States because of the lack of a single, uniform definition of sexual abuse and because few comprehensive studies have been conducted (Koss *et al.*, 1994). However, some data are available on the prevalence of sexual abuse of women in the general population and in samples of women with SPMI. These prevalence estimates vary greatly because of differences in the methodologies used to ascertain abuse and in the sample characteristics (e.g., ethnicity, social class and diagnosis).

In the general population, reports of rates of child sexual abuse range from approximately seven percent to 62%, with most researchers estimating prevalence in the range of 25% to 30% (Finkelhor, Hotaling, Lewis & Smith, 1990; Sandberg, Lynn & Green, 1994). Published rates of adult sexual assault are somewhat lower than those of childhood sexual abuse, ranging from 14% to 25% (National Victims Center, 1992; Wyatt, 1992). Reported rates of sexual abuse in studies of women with SPMI are higher than in the general population. For childhood sexual abuse, rates range from 20% to 73% with a median rate of 51%. Prevalence rates for adult sexual abuse in studies of women receiving mental health services range from 21% to 76% with a median rate of 33% (Goodman, Johnson, Dutton & Harris, 1997; Mueser *et al.*, in press). Studies combining childhood and adult sexual abuse have found rates of up to 76% among episodically homeless women with SPMI and rates of 51% in state hospital psychiatric patients (Craine, Henson, Colliver & MacLean, 1988; Goodman, Dutton & Harris, 1995).

The prevalence rates discussed previously are likely to be underestimates of the actual rates of sexual abuse in both general and SPMI samples. The bias towards underestimation may result both from sampling bias and other methodological artifacts. With regard to sampling, many studies did not include non-English speaking women, incarcerated women, or women without telephones, all of whom may be at especially high risk of abuse. In clinical settings, women who have experienced sexual abuse may be unlikely to disclose the abuse to a health worker and when they do disclose the abuse, they may under-report its frequency (Brown & Anderson, 1991).

In general, underreporting has been attributed to several factors. First, women may underreport abuse because of feelings of shame, guilt, or fear or because they want to protect the perpetrators (Della Femina, Yaeger & Lewis, 1990). Second, women may not disclose abuse because they are unsure how the health worker will respond and fear that the response will include horror, denial, or rejection (Symonds, 1982). Third, women may fail to report abuse simply because they fail to label the experience as abuse (Cascardi, Mueser, DeGirolomo & Murrin, 1996). Fourth, women may not disclose abuse because they wish to avoid discussing unpleasant memories (Dill, Chu & Grob, 1991). It has been hypothesized that African American survivors of sexual abuse in particular may be hesitant to disclose abuse because such issues have been traditionally interpreted as family matters not to be discussed with outsiders, particularly in cases of incest (Millett, 1997). Finally, some abuse survivors may experience amnesia for the abuse (Feldman-Summers & Pope, 1994) and thus not report.

On the other hand, it is possible that some of the studies cited provide prevalence estimates which exceed population rates. This may be due to several factors. First, many studies that examined the prevalence of sexual abuse used convenience samples, which could result in biased estimates. Second, it is possible that certain settings or disorders may be associated with disproportionately high rates of abuse. For example, a number of the published studies of women with severe mental illness have used inpatient samples, or clients with histories of homelessness. To the extent that past abuse increases illness severity or service utilization, reliance on samples of acute patients or high service utilizers may yield inflated estimates of abuse prevalence in the SPMI population. Third, some studies may have used less stringent criteria of abuse or did not carefully evaluate reports of abuse.

Sexual Abuse Correlates and Hypothesized Mechanisms

Sexual abuse has been associated with a wide range of hypothesized sequelae in the general population, including substance abuse and psychological disorders such as depression and borderline personality disorders (for a review, see Polusny & Follett, 1995). One of the most commonly reported correlates of sexual abuse is PTSD (Kessler, Sonnega, Bromet, Hugher & Nelson, 1995).

Research has also linked sexual abuse to psychological sequelae in women with SPMI (Muenzenmaier, Meyer, Struening & Ferber, 1993).

For example, Ross, Anderson and Clark (1994) studied the link between childhood physical and sexual abuse and symptoms of schizophrenia. They found that those with a history of child abuse were significantly more likely to report positive symptoms of schizophrenia. However, this study has not been replicated. Research has also linked childhood sexual abuse in SPMI samples to such diverse psychological symptoms as: sexual delusions, depression, major medical problems, somatization, interpersonal sensitivity, anxiety, paranoid ideation, borderline personality disorder, suicidal symptoms, and psychoticism (Beck & van der Kolk, 1987).

Additional correlates of childhood sexual abuse include coping deficits and increases in self-destructive behavior (Blankertz, Cnaan & Freedman, 1993). Although these deficits are found in women without SPMI, they can become magnified in women with SPMI, thus becoming extremely debilitating (Anderson & Chiocchio, 1997). Moreover, hospitalized women with SPMI and childhood sexual abuse histories are more likely to be secluded and restrained, require more staff time and receive more neuroleptics.

Episodically homeless women with SPMI and childhood abuse histories are more likely to experience adult victimization, to engage in prostitution, and to abuse substances (Goodman & Fallot, in press). Fewer studies have investigated the correlates of sexual abuse which occurred in adulthood. A study of episodically homeless women with SPMI (Goodman et al., 1995) examined victimization across the lifespan. They found that the recency of violence, the frequency of violence across the lifespan and child sexual abuse, were associated with a variety of psychiatric symptoms including hostility, anxiety, dissociation, depression, somatization, and PTSD symptoms. In sum, sexual abuse correlates include: 1) PTSD, 2) substance use disorders, 3) homelessness, 4) risky sexual behavior, and 5) revictimization.

These correlates are examined more closely in the following sections, including discussion of commonly hypothesized mechanisms linking abuse to these five variables. However, it is important to note that, in the absence of longitudinal data, it is difficult to tease apart causes and effects related to sexual abuse in women with SPMI. It is possible that sexual abuse leads to the psychological symptoms we have listed. It is equally possible that psychological disorders may lead to sexual abuse, due to increased vulnerability to victimization. In addition, it is possible that a third factor (e.g., substance abuse) may moderate the relationship between sexual abuse and psychological disorders. All of these hypotheses may be correct to different degrees, and for different sub-populations of women with SPMI.

1) **PTSD:** PTSD is a psychological disorder that results from experiencing or witnessing a traumatic event. The DSM-IV's (APA, 1994) definition of PTSD includes having "experienced, witnessed, or [been] confronted with an event or events that involved actual or threatened death or serious injury, or a threat to the physical integrity of others,

[and responding with intense fear, helplessness or horror]." (pp. 427–428). Symptoms include the reexperiencing of the traumatic event (i.e., through images, dreams, distress at exposure to cues that evoke the event), avoidance of stimuli associated with the trauma or psychic numbing, and increased arousal. Sexual abuse, occurring either in childhood or in adulthood, generally meets the traumatic event criterion for PTSD, and researchers have found that PTSD is a common long-term correlate of childhood sexual abuse (Kessler *et al.*, 1995).

The prevalence rate of PTSD in the general population has been estimated to be about eight to nine percent (Breslau, Davis, Andreski & Peterson, 1991). In nonclinical samples, the rate of PTSD in adults with histories of childhood sexual abuse is consistently greater than 65% (Davidson & Smith, 1990; O' Neill & Gupta, 1991). Sexual abuse in adulthood is associated with developing PTSD in 25% to 50% of women in nonclinical samples (Resnick, Kilpatrick, Dansky, Saunders & Best, 1993). Mueser *et al.* (in press) investigated the extent to which a range of traumatic events were related to PTSD in women with SPMI. They found that childhood sexual assault was the traumatic event most likely to be associated with PTSD, with an odds ratio of 4.73. Childhood sexual assault was closely followed by lifetime sexual assault (odds ratio 4.29) and adult sexual assault (odds ratio 2.77). However, only child sexual abuse and number of types of trauma experienced uniquely predicted PTSD in women with SPMI.

PTSD may be correlated with sexual abuse in women with SPMI for several reasons. First, SPMI may be a risk factor for adult abuse and PTSD. Serious mental disorders involve symptoms such as limited reality testing, planning difficulties, impaired judgment, and difficulty with social relationships. These symptoms may increase vulnerability to sexual abuse, which may lead to PTSD (Kelly *et al.*, 1992). A second way SPMI might be related to PTSD is that the traumatic incidents resulting in PTSD may either precipitate the onset of severe mental illness in vulnerable individuals, or the traumatic incidents may trigger relapses in women who already have a severe and persistent mental illness. Third, it is possible that sexual abuse survivors may be misdiagnosed as having a SPMI, such as schizophrenia, when, in fact, they would be more appropriately diagnosed as having PTSD. There have been a number of published studies which document the presence of psychotic symptoms, such as delusions, in severe PTSD, which could lead to such misdiagnosis. Finally, women with disorders such as depression might be more likely to remember past traumatic experiences, thus leading to PTSD symptoms secondary to their other symptoms (Goodman *et al.*, 1997; Mueser *et al.*, in press).

2) Substance use disorders: A traumatic abuse history, particularly child sexual abuse, has been shown to be a major risk factor for substance use disorders (Blankertz, Cnaan & Freedman, 1993; Nash, Hulsey, Sexton, Harralson & Lambert, 1993). Two studies of inpatient samples found that childhood sexual abuse was significantly related to substance abuse (Beck & van der Kolk, 1987; Craine *et al.*, 1988). Goodman and Fallot (in press) reported that, among SPMI women, those with histories of childhood sexual abuse were three and one half times more likely to abuse alcohol and four and one half times more likely to abuse cocaine. The relationship between substance use and sexual abuse may be a function of several factors. First, it is possible that sexual abuse survivors may abuse substances as a method of numbing or avoiding the pain of recollecting the abuse (Anderson & Chiocchio, 1997). Next, women may be abused in the process of obtaining or using illegal drugs (Goodman *et al.*, 1995). Third, substance use impairs judgment and reduces inhibitions which may result in risky behaviors or subsequent abuse. It is also possible that individuals whose parents are substance abusers may be more likely to be sexually abused and also more likely to develop substance abuse disorders.

3) **Homelessness:** Homelessness has been shown to be correlated with sexual abuse history (Browne, 1993; Feitel, Margetson, Chamas & Lipton, 1992). Homeless women report higher rates of sexual abuse than do members of the general population. Studies of samples of non-SPMI homeless women have found that up to 70% reported being sexually abused in childhood and up to 43% reported being attacked as adults, rates higher than those of the general population (D'Ercole & Sturening, 1990; North & Smith, 1992; Shinn, Knickman & Weitzman, 1991). In a sample of SPMI women, Goodman *et al.* (1995) found that 34% reported experiencing adult sexual assault during a period of homelessness. Anderson and Chiocchio (1997) believe that child and adult sexual and physical abuse may be the first experience in a process that culminates in homelessness for some individuals (p. 24).

Abuse may lead to or exacerbate depressive symptoms or the distrust of others (Briere, 1984), and thus lead to social isolation (Russell, 1986). The depression or social isolation resulting from abuse may serve to eliminate sources of support for poor women, thus increasing their vulnerability to homelessness (Goodman, 1991). Further, young women may choose to leave home in an attempt to escape an abusive home situation or be forced out after disclosing abuse. Homelessness and sexual abuse may also be correlated because homeless women are more likely to live in communities where levels of assault are high, protective resources are low, and opportunities for escape are limited (Browne, 1993). Thus, there may be multiple pathways from sexual abuse to homelessness. First, sexual abuse may lead to mental illness which may lead to homelessness. Second, sexual abuse may lead to social distress or avoidance which may lead to poor social supports and homelessness. Finally, sexual abuse may lead to homelessness as a method of escaping the abuse.

4) **Risky sexual behavior:** Research has shown that childhood sexual abuse increases the likelihood of risky sexual behaviors such as having multiple sexual partners, trading sex for drugs or money, or having sex with risky partners (e.g., Cunningham, Stiffman, Dore &

Earls, 1994). Goodman and Fallot (in press) found that among SPMI homeless women, child sexual abuse was significantly related to prostitution and marginally correlated with knowingly having sexual relations with risky (HIV positive or IV drug using) partners. The authors reported that women with sexual abuse histories were about six and one half times more likely to engage in prostitution and four times more likely to engage in risky sexual behaviors.

One possible mechanism linking sexual abuse to risky sexual behavior involves cognitions about the self that arise from early abuse experiences. Adult survivors frequently believe that their own needs are irrelevant when compared with others' demands, that their bodies are not their own, and that they are legitimate objects for sexual exploitation (Wyatt, Guthrie & Notgrass, 1992). However, other mechanisms are possible and need further investigation.

5) **Revictimization:** Studies have found that being exposed to abuse in childhood greatly increases the chances of other forms of abuse being present and repeated in adulthood (Gidycz, Hanson & Hayman, 1995; Rose, 1993). Goodman and Fallot (in press) found that episodically homeless, SPMI women who were sexually abused as children were three and one half times more likely to experience adult sexual abuse and one and one half times more likely to experience adult physical abuse. Mueser *et al.* (in press) examined the relationship between SPMI and revictimization. They found that SPMI patients who had been exposed to traumatic events at some point in their lives tended to have been multiply traumatized, with exposure to an average of three to four types of trauma.

What are the possible mechanisms linking revictimization with a prior history of sexual abuse? From an object relations perspective, early abuse experiences may lead victims to confuse or link nurturance and intimacy with victimization, especially when the abuser is a caretaker. From a social learning perspective, women who have been subjected to early abuse may lack adequate role models in regards to establishing personal boundaries, or in the development of social skills to avoid or manage risky situations. As discussed above, traumatic abuse has been correlated with substance abuse, often seen as a device to avoid remembering past traumatic events. Paradoxically, substance abuse may increase vulnerability to revictimization, bringing to mind Santayana's caution that "those who [seek to] forget the past are condemned to relive it."

Clinical Implications of Sexual Abuse History
in Women with SPMI

Clearly, service providers and systems of care for women with SPMI must recognize the elevated prevalence of sexual abuse, and common sequelae of abuse, when assessing, treating and helping to support their clients through episodes of illness and community tenure. Both clinical experience and research suggest that women often do not spontaneously disclose abuse to providers, although it may be experienced as one of the most salient issues in their lives. At the same time, women report themselves to be quite comfortable with disclosure when asked directly and professionally about past and current abuse; and such disclosure can improve trust and sense of alliance with the provider.

A history of sexual abuse may have an impact on the assessment and treatment of women with SPMI. Issues surrounding self-disclosure, alliance with service providers, special needs and vulnerabilities require particular sensitivity. Even assessing past trauma history and current sequelae in SPMI women requires a certain degree of awareness and skill on the part of the interviewer. For example, survivors of sexual abuse in general, and those who were abused by their caregivers or those with power over them in particular, might be less likely to trust service providers and thus less likely to disclose or discuss abuse histories with them (Jacobson & Richardson, 1987). It has been suggested that health workers should be careful to give survivors an explanation of the importance of obtaining this information and to allow survivors to control the pace and format of the interview (Brown & Anderson, 1991; Forster & King, 1994). Several researchers have observed that the health worker should be careful not to verbally denigrate or denounce abusers, because survivors frequently still have relationships with the abusers, or may have mixed feelings towards them (Comas-Diaz & Green, 1994; Spielvogel & Floyd, 1997). This may be especially pertinent in cases of domestic assault. While it is important to be receptive to reports of abuse and victimization, it is equally important that the health care worker respect clients' wishes not to talk about the abuse at a particular point in time.

Treatment participation and alliance: There is growing awareness that SPMI women with histories of abuse have particular needs and vulnerabilities which must be understood by their mental health treatment providers. These include needs for both objective and subjective safety from revictimization, heightened fears regarding coercion and restraint, needs for empowerment and sense of efficacy, and needs for being valued and respected by those in the treatment system. Particular efforts are required to provide these conditions for women whose life experience has made them fearful or pessimistic about the interpersonal world. Standard responses to self-destructive behaviors (involuntary hospitalization, use of restraints), although intended to provide safety for a client, can be experienced as retraumatization by women who have been sexually coerced or abusively confined. Even interactions in non-acute situations can be threatening or alienating to women with severe trauma histories. Harris, for example (1997), writes that case managers need to be aware of how their boundaries can affect sexual trauma survivors. She observes that being too flexible or informal may remind trauma survivors of when their interpersonal boundaries were violated. This can trigger confusion about the intentions of providers. Conversely, she cautions that case managers need to be aware of being too authoritarian or hierarchical which may serve to reenact elements of past abusive relationships.

A number of complexities have been noted by providers who have offered mental health services to homeless women with abuse histories. Shelter residents, for example, often lack privacy, control, and feelings of safety. Harris (1997) has argued for addressing these issues by allowing shelter residents to have their own rooms, bathrooms, or private space, by allowing them to choose when and where they will sleep, and by giving them control over the selection of their roommates. In this context, it is important for shelters to foster a sense of community between clients as well as between clients and the staff (Goodman *et al.*, 1997a).

It may be important for mental health workers to provide abuse survivors with psycho-educational interventions, including basic information about abuse such as prevalence rates, short and long-term sequelae of trauma, and treatment options for dealing with abuse sequelae (Harris, 1997). A primary hurdle health mental health workers must tackle when treating sexual abuse survivors with SPMI is that frequently survivors possess little or no knowledge about either sexual or physical abuse trauma and their consequences. Another immediate concern is often teaching trauma survivors how to assess current environmental threats, and how to protect themselves from actual danger. At the same time, Harris emphasizes that women need to understand that there are limits on their abilities to avoid random physical violence. Unfortunately, very little is now known about the efficacy of such interventions in women with SPMI, and this will be a vital area for future research.

Another potential hurdle that health workers must overcome is their lack of knowledge of the social context in which abuse survivors live (Goodman *et al.*, 1997a). These environments would challenge the coping skills of virtually anyone, and can be overwhelming for people with cognitive deficits, thought disorder and severe affective symptoms. This issue may be especially salient for homeless women with SPMI. Therefore, inquiries into the constant threat and danger with which these women live may help health workers to understand previously inexplicable behaviors and to shed new light on how clients attempt to cope, and how they perceive themselves and others (Goodman *et al.*, 1997a). To further complicate this issue, the problem of "secondary traumatization" can very much intrude on providers, both delimiting their ability to relate to clients' needs and disclosure of events, and affecting providers' own emotional well-being. These problems may be particularly salient when providers themselves are abuse survivors who may be vulnerable to re-experiencing and retraumatization when exposed to episodes similar to events in their own lives.

CONCLUSION

A significant proportion of women with SPMI have experienced, and/or continually face, the threat of violent victimization, particularly sexual assault. The sequelae of such events appear to include a variety of symptoms and behaviors. Indeed, the preliminary evidence suggests that PTSD in particular is so prevalent among women with SPMI that it represents a major category of comorbid psychiatric illness in this population. Although many clinicians working with women with SPMI, and mental health consumers themselves, are acutely aware of these problems, they have only recently begun to receive systematic attention. It appears that, as in the general population, the effects of abuse and violent victimization- both sexual and physical- are multifaceted, with likely effects on primary psychiatric symptoms, adjustment, social function, quality of life, high risk behaviors and revictimization. The mutual effects of severe psychiatric disorders and post-traumatic disorders represent an almost totally uncharted territory empirically, and many questions remain about the directionality of the observed correlations. Even the basic phenomenology of post-abuse symptoms in women with SPMI has not been well charted, nor compared to the course of post-traumatic disorders in the general population. In this sense, understanding post-traumatic disorders, as they affect women with SPMI, can be seen as analogous to the understanding of substance use disorders in this same population a decade or more ago. That is, the elevated comorbidity of substance use disorders (SUD) in people with SPMI came to be recognized in the psychiatric literature, and the toxic effects of the comorbid SUD were somewhat better understood and documented during the 80's and 90's (Drake, Rosenberg & Mueser, 1996; Regier et al., 1990). Consequently, systems of care became generally aware of and responsive to SPMI clients who also abused psychoactive substances (Drake & Mueser, 1996; Minkoff & Drake, 1989). Effective treatments were developed and tested which responded to the needs of clients suffering both disorders. Like SUD, PTSD appears to affect almost half of all people with SPMI; a rate approximately four times higher than the population as a whole. Like SUD a decade ago, PTSD is rarely diagnosed by clinicians treating people with SPMI (Cascardi et al., 1996; Mueser et al., in press). As in SUD, most mental health providers do not feel comfortable with or knowledgeable about sexual abuse and the treatment of its after-effects. Like SUD in the SPMI a decade ago, no empirically validated treatments exist for people with both disorders. While all these issues are complex, addressing them would also appear to represent a necessary step in providing meaningful care for women with severe and persistent mental illness who have also suffered sexual abuse.

REFERENCES

American Psychiatric Association (1994). *Diagnostic and Statistical Manual of Mental Disorders (Fourth Edition- Revised) (DSM-IV)*. Washington, DC: Author.

Anderson, C.M. & Chiocchio, K.B. (1997). The interface of homelessness, addictions and mental illness in the lives of trauma survivors. In Harris, M. & Landis, C.L. (Eds.): *Sexual Abuse in the Lives of Women Diagnosed with Serious Mental Illness*, pp. 21–38. Australia: Harwood Academic Publishers.

Beck, J.C. & van der Kolk, B.A. (1987). Reports of childhood incest and current behavior of chronicallly hospitalized psychotic women. *American Journal of Psychiatry* 144:1474–1476.

Blankertz, L.E., Cnaan, R.A. & Freedman, E. (1993). Childhood risk factors in dually diagnosed homeless adults. *Social Work* 38(5):587–595.

Breslau, N., Davis, G.C., Andreski, P. & Peterson, E. (1991). Traumatic events and posttraumatic stress disorder in an urban population of young adults. *Archives of General Psychiatry* 48:216–222.

Briere, J. (1984). The effects of childhood sexual abuse on later psychological functioning: Defining a post-sexual abuse syndrome. Presented to the Third National Conference on Sexual Victimization of Children, Washington, D.C.

Brown, G.R. & Anderson, B. (1991). Psychiatric morbidity in adult inpatients with childhood histories of sexual and physical abuse. *American Journal of Psychiatry* 148(1):55–61.

Browne, A. (1993). Family violence and homelessness: The relevance of trauma histories in the lives of homeless women. *American Journal of Orthopsychiatry* 63:370–384.

Cascardi, M., Mueser, K.T., DeGirolomo, J. & Murrin, M. (1996). Physical aggression against psychiatric inpatients by family members and partners: A descriptive study. *Psychiatric Services* 47:531–533.

Comaz-Diaz, L. & Green, B. (1994). *Women of Color: Integrating Ethnic and Gender Identities in Psychotherapy*: New York, Guilford Press.

Craine, L.S., Henson, C.E., Colliver, J.A. & MacLean, D.G. (1988). Prevalence of a history of sexual abuse among female psychiatric patients in a state hospital system. *Hospital and Community Psychiatry* 39(3):300–304.

Cunningham, R.M., Stiffman, A.R., Dore, P. & Earls, F. (1994). The association of physical and sexual abuse with HIV risk behavior in adolescence and young adulthood: Implications for public health. *Child Abuse and Neglect* 18(3):233–245.

Davidson, J. & Smith, R. (1990). Traumatic experiences in psychiatric outpatients. *Journal of Traumatic Stress* 3:459–475.

Della Femina, D., Yaeger, C. & Lewis, D. (1990). Child abuse: Adolescent records vs. adult recall. *Child Abuse and Neglect* 14(2):227–231.

D'Ercole, A. & Struening, E. (1990). Victimization among homeless women: Implications for service delivery. *Journal of Community Psychology* 18: 141–152.

Dill, D., Chu, J. & Grob, M. (1991). The reliability of abuse history reports: A comparison of two inquiry formats. *Comprehensive Psychiatry* 32(2): 166–9.

Drake, R.E. & Mueser, K.T. (1996). *New Directions for Mental Health Services*. San Francisco: Jossey-Bass.

Drake, R.E., Rosenberg, S.D. & Mueser, K.T. (1996). Assessment of substance use disorders in person with severe mental illness. In Drake, R.E. & Mueser, K.T. (Eds.): *New Directions for Mental Health Services.* San Francisco: Jossey-Bass.

Feitel, B., Margetson, N., Chamas, J. & Lipton, C. (1992). Psychosocial background and behavioral and emotional disorders of homeless and runaway youth. *Hospital and Community Psychiatry* 43:155–159.

Feldman-Summers, S. & Pope, K.S. (1994). The experience of forgetting childhood abuse: A national survey of psychologists. *Journal of Consulting and Clinical Psychology* 62(3):636–9.

Finkelhor, D., Hotaling, G., Lewis, I.A. & Smith, C. (1990). Sexual abuse in a national survey of adult men and women: Prevalence, characteristics, and risk factors. *Child Abuse and Neglect* 14:19–28.

Forster, P. & King, J. (1994). Traumatic stress reactions and the psychiatric emergency. *Psychiatric Annals* 24(11):603–614.

Gidycz, Hanson & Layman. (1995). A prospective analysis of the relationships among sexual assault experiences. *Psychology of Women Quarterly,* 19:5–29.

Goodman, L.A. (1991). The prevalence of abuse among homeless and housed poor mothers: A comparison study. *American Journal of Orthopsychiatry* 6(14):489–500.

Goodman, L.A., Dutton, M.A. & Harris, M. (1995). Physical and sexual assault prevalence among episodically homeless women with serious mental illness. *American Journal of Orthopsychiatry* 65(4):468–478.

Goodman, L.A. & Fallott, R. (in press). The association of physical and sexual abuse with HIV risk behaviors and revictimization in episodically homeless, mentally ill women. *American Journal of Orthopsychiatry.*

Goodman, L.A., Johnson, M., Dutton, M.A. & Harris, M. (1997a). Prevalence and impact of sexual and physical abuse in women with severe mental illness. In Harris, M. & Landis, C.L. (Eds.): *Sexual Abuse in the Lives of Women Diagnosed with Serious Mental Illness,* pp. 277–299. Australia: Harwood Academic Publishers.

Goodman, L.A., Rosenberg, S.D., Mueser, K.T. & Drake, R.E. (1997b). Physical and sexual assault history in women with serious mental illness: Prevalence, impact, treatment, and future research directions. *Schizophrenia Bulletin* 23(4):685–696.

Harris, M. (1997). Modifications in service delivery for women diagnosed with severe mental illness who are also the survivors of sexual abuse trauma. In Harris, M. & Landis, C.L. (Eds.): *Sexual Abuse in the Lives of Women Diagnosed with Serious Mental Illness* pp. 3-20. Australia: Harwood Academic Publishers.

Jacobson, A. & Richardson, B. (1987). Assault experiences of 100 psychiatric inpatients: Evidence of the need for routine inquiry. *American Journal of Psychiatry* 144:908–913.

Kelly, J.A., Murphy, D.A., Bahr, G.R., Brasfield, T.L., Davis, D.R., Hauth, A.C., Morgan, M.G., Stevenson, L.Y. & Eilers, M.K. (1992). AIDS/HIV risk behavior among the chronic mentally ill. *American Journal of Psychiatry* 149(7):886–9.

Kessler, R.C., Sonnega, A., Bromet, E., Hugher, M. & Nelson, C.B. (1995). Posttraumatic stress disorder in the national comorbidity survey. *Archives of General Psychiatry* 52:1048–1060.

Koss, M.P., Goodman, L.A., Browne, A., Fitzgerald, L.F., Keita, G.P. & Russo, N.F. (1994). *No safe haven: Male violence against women at home, at work, and in the community.* Washington, DC: American Psychological Association Press.

Millett, B.L. (1997). Sexual trauma and African American women. In Harris, M. & Landis, C.L. (Eds.): *Sexual Abuse in the Lives of Women Diagnosed with Serious Mental Illness* pp. 321–336. Australia: Harwood Academic Publishers.

Minkoff, K. & Drake, R. (Eds.): (1991). *Dual Diagnosis of Major Mental Illness and Substance Disorder.* San Francisco: Jossey-Bass.

Muenzenmaier, K., Meyer, I., Struening, E. & Ferber, J. (1993). Childhood abuse and neglect among women outpatients with chronic mental illness. *Hospital and Community Psychiatry* 44(7):666–670.

Mueser, K.T., Goodman, L.A., Trumbetta, S.L., Rosenberg, S.D., Osher, F.C., Vidaver, R.M., Auciello, P. & Foy, D.W. (in press). Trauma and posttraumatic stress disorder in severe mental illness. *Journal of Consulting and Clinical Psychology.*

Nash, M., Hulsey, T., Sexton, M., Harralson, T. & Lambert, W. (1993). Long-term sequelae of childhood sexual abuse: Perceived family environment, psychopathology and dissociation. *Journal of Consulting and Clinical Psychology* 61(2):276–283.

National Victims Center (1992). *Rape in America: A report to the nation.* Arlington, VA: Author.

North, C.S. & Smith, E.M. (1992). PTSD among homeless men and women. *Hospital and Community Psychiatry* 43(10):1010–1016.

O' Neill, K. & Gupta, K. (1991). Post-traumatic stress disorder in women who were victims of childhood sexual abuse. *Irish Journal of Psychological Medicine* 8:124–127.

Polusny, M.A. & Follette, V.M. (1995). Long-term correlates of child sexual abuse: Theory and review of the empirical literature. *Applied and Preventive Psychology* 4:143–166.

Regier, D.S., Farmer, M.E., Rae, D.S., Locke, B., Keith, S., Judd, L. & Goodwin, F. (1990). Comorbidity of mental disorders with alcohol and other drug abuse. *Journal of the American Medical Association* 264:2511–2518

Resnick, H.S., Kilpatrick, D.G., Dansky, B.S., Saunders, B.E. & Best, C.L. (1993). Prevalence of civilian trauma and post-traumatic stress disorder in a representative national sample of women. *Journal of Consulting and Clinical Psychology* 61:984–991.

Rose, D. (1993). Sexual assault, domestic violence and incest. In Stewart, D. & Stotland, N. (Eds.): *Psychological Aspects of Women's Health Care* pp. 447–483. Washington, D.C.: American Psychiatric Press.

Ross, C.A., Anderson, G. & Clark, P. (1994). Childhood abuse and the positive symptoms of schizophrenia. *Hospital and Community Psychiatry* 45:489–491.

Russell, D.E.H. (1986). *The secret trauma: Incest in the lives of girls and women.* New York: Basic.

Sandberg, D., Lynn, S.J. & Green, J.P. (1994). Sexual abuse and revictimization. In Lynn, S.J. & Rhue, J.W. (Eds.): *Dissociation.* New York, Guilford Press.

Shinn, M., Knickman, J. & Weitzman, B.C. (1991). Social relationships and vulnerability to becoming homeless among poor families. *American Psychologist* 46(11):1180–7.

Spielvogel, A.M. & Floyd, A.K. (1997). Assessment of trauma in women psychiatric patients. In Harris, M. & Landis, C.L. (Eds.): *Sexual Abuse in the Lives of Women Diagnosed with Serious Mental Illness* pp. 39–64. Australia: Harwood Academic Publishers.

Symonds, M. (1982). Victim responses to terror: Understanding and treatment. In Ochberg, F. & Soskis, D. (Eds.): *Victims of Terrorism.* Boulder, C.O.: Westview Press.

Wyatt, G.E. (1992). The sociocultural context of African American and White American women's rape. *Journal of Social Issues* 48:77–92.

Wyatt, G.E., Guthrie, D. & Notgrass, C. (1992). Differential effects of women's child sexual abuse and subsequent sexual revictimization. *Journal of Consulting and Clinical Psychology* 60:167–173.

9

Psychotropic Medications and Sexual Dysfunction

KAREN MILNER, RAJIV TANDON, OLADAPO TOMORI and TIMOTHY FLORENCE

INTRODUCTION

Reduction in sexual desire and performance are frequently reported by patients with various psychiatric disorders. Sexual dysfunction can also be induced by all classes of psychotropic medication. Distinguishing illness-associated sexual dysfunction from that induced by medications can be extremely difficult. Patients are apt to ascribe any reduction in sexual desire or inadequacy in sexual performance that they experience to the adverse effects of the prescribed medication, whereas the treating mental health professional is equally likely to attribute such sexual dysfunction to the patient's illness. The considerable clinical significance of the sexual dysfunction associated with psychotropic medications and the inadequate attention paid to this problem by treating physicians is illustrated by the following study. In 1990, Finn, Bailey, Schultz & Faber asked 41 patients with schizophrenia being treated with neuroleptics to rate the relative discomfort of symptoms and the side effects of the neuroleptics. A group of psychiatrists was asked to make parallel ratings from the perspective of the patient. Twenty side effects (i.e., akathisia, dystonia, dry mouth, orthostatic hypotension, impotence, inhibited/painful ejaculation, etc.) and 19 symptoms (i.e., persecutory delusions, thought blocking, auditory hallucinations, etc.) were rated. Overall, genital/sexual side effects were rated by the patients as the most bothersome of the symptoms or side effects; impotence was more bothersome than any of the schizophrenic symptoms. Although psychiatrists predicted patients' ratings moderately well, they misjudged the discomfort to patients of side effects and symptoms overall. Given this discrepancy, it is no surprise that compliance becomes an issue for many patients. The chapter by Deegan (Chapter 2) also provides clear testimony to the importance of this side-effect.

In this chapter, the physiology of sexual function is first reviewed and general concepts related to medication-induced sexual side effects summarized. Then the clinical management of sexual dysfunction relative to each class of psychotropic medication is discussed, with the objective of developing strategies to minimize or reverse these side effects. It is hoped that employment of the strategies suggested will not only increase treatment compliance, but also enhance the quality of life of the patients we serve.

THE SEXUAL RESPONSE CYCLE

A sequence of physiological responses typically occurs in response to sexual stimulation. This sequence of responses, termed the sexual response cycle, can be divided into four phases: desire, excitement, orgasm, and resolution (see Table 9.1). In the phase of sexual desire, a desire for sexual activity is engendered by visual, olfactory, or tactile sensations and/or fantasy. Impaired desire or hypoactive sexual

Table 9.1. Phases of the Sexual Response Cycle.

Phase 1. Desire–In this phase, the desire for sexual desire is engendered by visual, olfactory, or tactile sensations and/or fantasy.

Phase 2. Excitement–This phase consists of a subjective sense of sexual pleasure and the accompanying physiological changes. In men, this consists of penile tumescence and erection. In women, the changes involve vasocongestion in the pelvis, vaginal lubrication and expansion, and swelling of the external genitalia.

Phase 3. Orgasm–In this phase, sexual pleasure peaks, with release of sexual tension and rhythmic contraction of the perineal muscles and reproductive organs. In men, there is a sense of ejaculatory inevitability, which is followed by ejaculation of semen. In women, there are contractions of the wall of the outer third of the vagina.

Phase 4. Resolution–This phase in characterized by muscular relaxation and a sense of general well-being. During this phase, males are physiologically refractory to further erection and orgasm for a variable period of time. The post-orgasmic refractory period is absent in women, resulting in the potential for experiencing multiple orgasms.

desire disorder is the most common dysfunction of this aspect of sexual behavior.

In the excitement stage, a subjective sense of sexual pleasure is experienced. Accompanying physiological changes involve pelvic vasocongestion with accompanying myotonia. In men, this results in penile tumescence and erection; in women, vaginal lubrication, and expansion and swelling of the external genitalia. Erectile disorder in males and impaired sexual arousal and dyspareunia in females are examples of dysfunction of this phase of sexual response.

In the orgasmic phase, sexual pleasure peaks in association with rhythmic contraction of the perineal muscles and reproductive organs, cardiovascular and respiratory changes, and a release of sexual tension. In the male, there is the sensation of ejaculatory inevitability, which is followed by ejaculation of semen. In the female, there are contractions of the wall of the outer third of the vagina. Premature ejaculation in males and impaired orgasm in women are examples of dysfunction of this component of sexual response.

The resolution phase is characterized by muscular relaxation and a sense of well-being. Men experience a physiologic refractory period before erection and orgasm can occur again. The post-orgasmic refractory period is absent in women, resulting in the potential for experiencing multiple orgasms. Post-coital headache and post-coital dysphoria are examples of disturbances in this aspect of the sexual response cycle.

THE BIOLOGY OF SEXUAL FUNCTIONING

The understanding of the biology underlying the sexual response cycle is not yet complete. Much of what we know is derived from animal models or analysis of the effect of disease or medication on human sexual functioning. Additionally, most studies have focused on male erection and ejaculation with results generalized to women. However, it is clear that sexual functioning involves a complex interplay of neurotransmitters, hormones, and peptides, acting both centrally and peripherally (Crenshaw & Goldberg, 1996; Gitlin, 1994; Schiavi and Schreiner-Engel, 1980; Seagraves, 1989). An overview of the present state of our knowledge is summarized below.

Brain Localization of Sexual Functioning

Sexual functioning is localized to different areas of the brain. The frontal and cerebral cortices process sensory information and cognitive thought, as well as "learning, memory and emotional reactions". Subcortical structures (i.e., limbic system, basal ganglia, and pituitary gland) "mediate reflexive and vegetative functions as well as hormonal and neuropeptide activity" (Crenshaw & Goldberg, 1996).

Neurotransmitters and Sexual Function

Evidence from both animal and human studies suggests that dopamine is associated with the erectile response in humans. This response appears to be centrally mediated given that it can be inhibited by central, but not peripheral, dopamine blockers. It has been speculated that the site of this activity is the nucleus accumbens. In rats, the nucleus accumbens is the site at which intentions, thoughts, habitual actions, and emotional reflexes are translated into purposeful activity. Alternatively, dopamine may exert its central effect via a stimulatory effect on oxytocin. Augmented sexual activity has been noted with dopamine agonists; likewise, decreased libido and erectile dysfunction have been associated with dopamine blockers, such as the conventional neuroleptics.

Adrenergic mechanisms are integrally involved in both erection and ejaculation. Centrally, adrenergic activity increases arousal generally via release of norepinephrine from the locus coeruleus. Peripherally, penile detumescence (vasoconstriction) appears to be mediated by both $alpha_1$ and $alpha_2$ stimulation. Peripheral alpha adrenergic blockade obstructs venous outflow from the corpora cavernosa, resulting in prolonged erection. Therefore, medications with alpha adrenergic blocking activity will promote erection, and, in extreme cases, priapism particularly when unopposed by cholinergic blockade. $Alpha_1$ adrenergic function is also involved in ejaculation; agents with $alpha_1$ antagonist properties (i.e., conventional antipsychotics, tricyclics, etc.) can cause ejaculatory dysfunction.

The role of serotonin in sexual arousal or erection is predominantly inhibitory. Enhanced central serotonergic function results in decreased dopaminergic functioning with a consequent decrease in libido. Clinically, treatment with serotonin reuptake inhibitors (SSRIs) can result in decreased libido, erectile dysfunction, ejaculatory disturbance, delayed orgasm, and anorgasmia. Central mechanisms appear to be involved in that treatment with cyproheptadine, an antihistamine with antiserotonergic properties, is associated with a return of sexual functioning in some patients taking a serotonergic antidepressant. Interestingly, buspirone, a serotonin agonist, causes an increase in sexual activity, most probably via its selective activity at the $5HT_{1A}$ receptor. Peripherally, serotonergic innervation may contribute to decreased orgasmic functioning as well as penile anesthesia.

Centrally, acetylcholine mediates "sexual thoughts, attitudes, and memories" via its activity in the limbic system (Crenshaw & Goldberg, 1996). Stimulation of parasympathetic pathways (second and third sacral roots) elicits penile erection. Acetylcholine is the neurotransmitter in the parasympathetic ganglia as well as in the parasympathetic innervation of the penile blood vessels and corporeal trabecular smooth muscles. However, atropine produces inconsistent effects on erectile function; therefore it is likely that erection is mediated via cholinergic activity in association with activity of some other neurotransmitter or neuropeptide. Cholinergic activity also clearly has an important indirect role in maintaining adrenergic-cholinergic balance. Priapism may be associated with alpha blocking agents, particularly in the absence of anticholinergic activity. Peripheral cholinergic activity also promotes secretory processes involved in sexual activity (i.e., anticholinergic activity results in drying of the mucous membranes).

Antagonism of histaminergic activity centrally may result in sedation, decreased cutaneous sensitivity, and reduced secretions. The inhibitory effects of GABA are also centrally mediated and result in decreased arousal via sedation and cognitive impairment. Neurotransmitter effect is summarized in Table 9.2.

Hormones and Sexual Function

Luteinizing hormone (LH) and follicle-stimulating hormone (FSH) are synthesized and released from the pituitary gland in response to a hypothalamic releasing factor or hormone (variously called gonadotropin-releasing hormone [GnRH], LHRH, or luteinizing hormone releasing factor [LRF]). In women, luteinizing hormone (LH) controls ovulation and the formation and maintenance of the corpus luteum via effects on estrogen and progesterone. Follicle stimulating hormone (FSH) controls the growth and maturation of the ovarian follicle. In men, LH triggers production and secretion of testosterone and dihydrotestosterone in the Leydig cells, which maintain male genital and accessory organ tissues and promote male sex behavior. FSH controls sperm production, maintains the seminiferous tubules, and participates in stimulation of Leydig cell testosterone production.

The secretion of LH and FSH is relatively constant in men, but varies greatly in women during the menstrual cycle. At the beginning of the menstrual cycle, LH and FSH secretion are increased in response to low circulating levels of estrogen. Follicular development follows, as does an increase in the plasma concentration of estrogen. One follicle becomes dominant and begins to secrete large amounts of estrogen. The increase in estrogen levels triggers a short secretory peak of LH and FSH at the mid-point of the menstrual cycle. The mid-cycle surge of

Table 9.2. Neurotransmitter Effect on Sexual Function.

Excitatory	Inhibitory
Dopamine	Serotonin
Norepinephrine	GABA
Acetylcholine	
Histamine	

LH induces ovulation and results in formation of the corpus luteum, which secretes large amounts of both estrogen and progesterone. This, in turn, suppresses the activity of the hypothalamus and pituitary, resulting in low circulating levels of LH and FSH. Inhibin, a hormone secreted by the corpus luteum, is also elevated during the luteal phase and contributes to the suppression of FSH secretion. In unfertilized cycles, plasma estrogen and progesterone levels drop, with degeneration of the corpus luteum and menstruation (Vander, Sherman & Luciano, 1994).

In addition to feedback inhibition of GNRH secretion by the hypothalamus and LH secretion by the anterior pituitary, estrogen and testosterone are involved in fetal differentiation and growth, differential induction of the secondary sexual characteristics, and gametogenesis. As regards sexual functioning, estrogens facilitate all stages of the sexual response cycle in women (i.e., desire, attraction, lubrication, orgasm, and satisfaction), and promote the action of serotonin, opioids, prolactin, and oxytocin. Their effects on male sexuality are unclear (Crenshaw & Goldberg, 1996).

Testosterone promotes sex drive, assertiveness, and aggressiveness in both sexes. In men, it promotes orgasm and ejaculation. In women, it stimulates interest in genital sex and enhances the drive for orgasm; hence, masturbation is sought more than intercourse. This contrasts with the effect of estrogen which stimulates the receptive sex drive. The receptive sex drive is associated with a woman's desire for penetration and motivates her to have sex with a partner rather than masturbate. In both sexes, testosterone facilitates the stimulatory activity of dopamine and epinephrine, and is inhibitory to serotonin, opioids, and prolactin (Crenshaw & Goldberg, 1996). Testosterone also weakly inhibits monoamine oxidase resulting in mild antidepressant activity.

Progesterone has feedback effects at both the hypothalamus and the pituitary. In addition, it functions to ready the uterine environment for implantation via its effects on glandular tissue and uterine contractility. Prior to birth, it stimulates growth of the glandular tissue in the breast and inhibits the milk-inducing effects of prolactin. Sexually, it is a deterrent to a woman's sexual functioning. Nurturant activities are promoted instead (i.e., cuddling and holding are sought in preference to genital stimulation). It has therefore been described as protective of maternal or mothering behaviors. Progesterone also inhibits sexual desire in men. In both sexes desire and sensitivity may also be indirectly inhibited by progesterone's facilitation of monoamine oxidase activity.

In women, prolactin stimulates breast development and milk production in response to increased estrogen levels prior to parturition. Artificially increased levels of prolactin can result in gynecomastia and galactorrhea in both men and women. Increased levels of prolactin can also decrease testosterone to below normal levels, resulting in inhibition of the sex drive; chronically increased levels of prolactin can lead to impotence. It is unclear whether the inhibition of the sex drive is a direct effect of prolactin or secondary to its effect on testosterone levels. At normal levels, prolactin may potentiate the stimulatory effects of LH on Leydig cells and of testosterone on its target cells. Hormonal effects on sexual functioning are summarized in Table 9.3.

Neuropeptides and Sexual Functioning

Oxytocin plays a role in both parturition and suckling. It is an extremely potent stimulant of uterine muscle both via a direct action on uterine smooth muscle and indirectly via its effect on the synthesis of prostaglandins, which also facilitate uterine contractions. Oxytocin is reflexly released as a result of input to the hypothalamus from receptors in the uterus, particularly the cervix. During pregnancy the concentration of oxytocin receptors in the uterus markedly and progressively increases as a result of estrogen stimulation and possibly, uterine distention. Contractions most likely occur as a result of uterine sensitivity to oxytocin, as well as a drop in estrogen and progesterone. Oxytocin is also involved in suckling via facilitation of contraction of the myoepithelial cells surrounding the alveoli of the breast (Vander, Sherman & Luciano, 1994).

Oxytocin's role is not limited to labor and nursing. Oxytocin increases during sexual activity in both men and women, with a spike during orgasm. The effect this has on sexual functioning in humans is unclear; however, in animals, oxytocin appears to activate erection by triggering a circuit through the cholinergic limbic system to the dopaminergic hypothalamus to the pituitary and into the spinal cord. In women, oxytocin is released in response to cervical and vaginal distention not only during labor and delivery, but also during sexual activity. Tactile sensitivity and grooming during and after a sexual encounter, as well as during parental behavior (for men also) and nursing/suckling are all potentiated by oxytocin. Thus, oxytocin may mediate behavior along a continuum from sexual activity to nursing and parenting (Crenshaw & Goldberg, 1996).

Vasopressin is an antidiuretic hormone that prevents water and salt depletion by stimulating thirst and inhibiting urination. It affects sexual functioning in both men and women via potentiation of

Table 9.3. Hormonal Effect on Sexual Function.

Excitatory	Inhibitory
Luteinizing Hormone Releasing Hormone (LHRH)	Estrogens (in men)
	Progesterone
Estrogens (in women)	Prolactin
Testosterone	

cholinergic activity in the limbic system. In men, its activity is linked to the presence of testosterone, suggesting modulation of male sexual behavior. It also appears to have a role in thermoregulation in men, preventing "overheating" of the brain areas involved in sexual activity (Crenshaw & Goldberg, 1996).

Vasoactive intestinal peptide (VIP) is a naturally occurring peptide neurotransmitter found in abundant quantities in the genitals of both sexes, the gastrointestinal tract, and the spinal cord. It is co-localized with acetylcholine peripherally, and "mediates vascular and smooth muscle relaxation" previously thought to be the sole function of the cholinergic input (Crenshaw & Goldberg, 1996). Its absence has been associated with impotence. Neuropeptide effects on sexual functioning are summarized in Table 9.4.

Table 9.4. Neuropeptide Effect on Sexual Function.

Excitatory
Oxytocin
Vasopressin
Vasoactive Intestinal Peptide (VIP)

MEDICATION-INDUCED SEXUAL DYSFUNCTION

Range of Medication-Induced Sexual Dysfunction

Sexual dysfunction may occur across the entire sexual response cycle. Psychotropic medication can result in alteration in sexual desire, orgasmic disorders, dyspareunia, infertility, and breast disorders in both sexes. In addition, psychotropic medication may result in lubrication disorders, menstrual disorders, and clitoral hypertrophy in women, and erection/arousal abnormalities and ejaculation disorders in both sexes. Decreased sexual desire, or hyposexuality, is the most common type of sexual dysfunction. It is frequently under-reported, both because patients attribute it to other causes (i.e., stress at work, etc.) and because physicians fail to elicit it. Antipsychotics are most frequently associated with decreased libido. The mechanism of action involves dopaminergic blockade, which results in increased prolactin or decreased testosterone levels. Antidepressants, benzodiazepines, and lithium can also cause decreased sexual desire. Erectile difficulty is the second most common sexual side effect of prescription drugs, followed by orgasmic difficulties in both men and women. Heterocyclic antidepressants, monoamine oxidase inhibitors (MAOIs), and neuroleptics (particularly when given in conjunction with an anticholinergic medication) are most likely to be associated with erectile dysfunction. Selective serotonin reuptake inhibitors (SSRIs) and MAOIs are most often associated with ejaculatory or orgasmic dysfunction, although neuroleptics and heterocyclic antidepressants have been implicated as well.

Mechanisms Underlying Medication-Induced Sexual Dysfunction

Gitlin (1994) has described four different mechanisms by which psychotropic medication can affect sexual functioning (see Table 9.5). The central nervous system can be affected directly or indirectly. Direct, or specific, sexual side effects occur when the medication alters neurotransmitter function (i.e., when SSRI-induced increase in serotonin results in decreased libido via effects on dopaminergic function). The central nervous system is affected indirectly when nonspecific effects of a medication result in general loss of sexual interest or functioning (i.e., when nausea secondary to an SSRI results in physical discomfort and decreased desire). Sexual functioning can also be affected peripherally, at the end organ. For example, alpha adrenergic blockade can result in prolonged erection or priapism. Finally, sexual dysfunction can occur as a result of hormonal changes that can occur in response to medication (i.e., when dopamine blockade results in increased prolactin production).

Frequency of Medication-Induced Sexual Dysfunction

Accurate estimates of medication-induced sexual dysfunction are difficult to obtain because most patients fail to report them and many clinicians fail to inquire about them. Case reports, brief case series, and a few controlled studies provide very approximate estimates of the frequency of this problem. Antihypertensives are the class of medication

Table 9.5. Mechanisms Underlying Medication-Induced Sexual Dysfunction.

Direct CNS Effects (i.e., SSRI-induced increase in serotonin results in decreased libido via effects on dopaminergic function).

Indirect CNS Effects (i.e., nausea secondary to a SSRI results in physical discomfort and decreased desire).

Peripheral Effects (i.e., alpha adrenergic blockade can result in prolonged erection or priapism).

Hormonal Effects (i.e., dopamine blockade results in increased prolactin production).

---

most frequently associated with medication-induced sexual dysfunction. In a study of the frequency of sexual dysfunction in a sample of patients receiving antihypertensives (DeLeo & Magni, 1983), spontaneous reporting of impotence was only 10% increasing to 26% on systematic oral questioning and 47% when completing a questionnaire. In general, psychiatric patients, particularly patients suffering from schizophrenia, are even less likely to spontaneously complain of sexual dysfunction. On the other hand, sexual dysfunction noted in patients receiving psychotropic medication may not be medication-induced; it could be idiosyncratic, associated with the psychiatric illness itself, associated with some concurrent medical illness, or be secondary to alcoholism or smoking that are often noted in patients with psychiatric illness. The relationship between psychotropic medication and sexual dysfunction is further obscured by the frequent absence of reliable information about baseline sexual function.

Detection and Differential Diagnosis of Medication-Induced Sexual Dysfunction

A careful history of the presenting complaint and factors that contribute to or mitigate its presence must be obtained to detect and diagnose medication-induced sexual dysfunction. Current concerns should be elicited, and baseline sexual functioning prior to the development of the psychiatric illness and following the development of the psychiatric illness but prior to the point that the medication was started must be elicited. Each phase of the sexual response cycle should be explored systematically. Questions involving the frequency of sexual intercourse, changes in frequency, date of last encounter, enjoyment, difficulty lubricating/becoming erect, ability to get and keep an erection, differential response to stimuli (i.e., inability to achieve an erection with a partner despite nocturnal emissions, ability to achieve orgasm via masturbation but not with partner, etc.), time to reach orgasm, difficulty reaching orgasm, changes in the quality of orgasm, dyspareunia, etc. should be raised. The presence of other psychiatric disorders, alcohol/substance abuse, or comorbid medical illnesses should be explored, and a list obtained of other medications being taken. Finally, the interpersonal context (i.e., relationship difficulties, job stress) in which the sexual dysfunction has arisen should be elicited (Crenshaw & Goldberg, 1996; Gitlin, 1994).

The differential diagnosis of medication-induced sexual dysfunction is extensive (see Table 9.6). Sexual dysfunction causally may be attributed to the presenting psychiatric disorder. For example, decreased sexual interest is a frequent complaint in those with major depressive disorder. Sexual dysfunction may also result from a comorbid psychiatric disorder (i.e., vaginismus, etc.). Medical illness can cause dysfunction in any phase of the sexual response cycle either directly or indirectly. For example, diabetic neuropathy may result in an inability

Table 9.6. Conditions or Disorders Associated with Sexual Dysfunction.

Endocrine	Immunological	Urological
Acromegaly	AIDS/HIV	Chronic kidney
Adrenal dysfunction	Arthritis	disease
Diabetes mellitus	Cancer	Cystitis
Hyperprolactinemia	Respiratory diseases	Epididymitis
Hypogonadism	**Neurological**	Peyronie's
Pituitary dysfunction	Alzheimer's disease	disease
Thyroid dysfunction	Brain lesions	Priapism
Gastrointestinal	Dementia	Prostatitis
Constipation/	Epilepsy	Renal failure
diarrhea	Multiple sclerosis	Urethrocele/
Irritable bowel	Parkinson's disease	cystocele
syndrome	Spinal cord injury/tumor	Urinary
Ulcerative colitis	Stroke	incontinence
Gynecological	**Psychiatric**	**Vascular**
Dysfunctional	Adjustment disorder	Arteriosclerosis
bleeding	Dysthymic disorder	Fistula
Dyspareunia	Generalized anxiety	Hypertension
Endometriosis	disorder	Ischemia
Genital Warts	Major depressive disorder	Myocardial
Infertility/pregnancy	Obsessive-compulsive	infarction
Menopause	disorder	TIA's
PMS	Posttraumatic stress	Venous
Vaginismus	disorder	insufficiency
Vaginitis	Schizophrenia	
	Somatization disorder	
	Specific phobia	
	Substance-induced disorder	

to achieve erection. A woman with endometriosis may experience pain upon penetration. Unpleasant physical sensations (i.e., nausea, lethargy, abdominal discomfort, etc.) that occur secondary to medical illness may result in apathy or lack of desire. Alcohol, illicit substances, and other medications also may affect sexual functioning adversely.

MEDICATION CLASSES AND SEXUAL DYSFUNCTION

Antipsychotics

Conventional antipsychotics or neuroleptics: In a 1987 study by Lingjaerde, Ahlfors, Bech, Dencker, and Elgen, psychiatrists from 50 hospitals in Scandinavia were asked to survey patients taking antipsychotics using the UKU side-effect rating scale. Two thousand three hundred and ninety-one patients were assessed (1,259 men and 1,132 women). Fifty-eight percent were being treated for schizophrenia. Most had been on the same agent for a number of years. Side effects were judged for severity (mild, moderate, severe) and supposed drug-relatedness (improbable, possible, probable). The occurrence of sexual side effects reported is listed in Table 9.7. Sexual dysfunction increased up to six months after first starting neuroleptic treatment and persisted unabated thereafter. Dysfunction was less pronounced in those taking higher potency, lower dose neuroleptics.

This survey illustrates the range of side effects attributable to the conventional antipsychotics. Similar findings have been documented in other studies. Thioridazine, particularly, has been associated with ejaculatory inhibition or retrograde ejaculation. The higher prevalence of sexual dysfunction attributed to both thioridazine and chlorpromazine may be due to anticholinergic and sedative actions.

Neuroleptics inhibit sexual functioning via several different mechanisms. The primary mechanism appears to be centrally mediated dopamine blockade, resulting in inhibition of function across the sexual response cycle. Secondarily, because dopamine inhibits the production of prolactin, dopamine blockade results in elevated levels of prolactin. In both men and women, elevated levels of prolactin can result in decreased desire and arousal. It is not clear whether this occurs directly or via the subsequent fall in testosterone and LHRH. In women, amenorrhea or menstrual irregularities may result, and in men spermatogenesis may be impaired. Galactorrhea, gynecomastia, and breast discomfort may occur in both sexes.

Sexual dysfunction related to the neuroleptics may also occur peripherally, as a result of alpha adrenergic blockade. As noted above, blockade can result in prolonged erection or priapism, particularly in the absence of corresponding anticholinergic activity. Cholinergic blockade in the limbic system may result in decreased arousal and impaired orgasm.

Indirect side effects attributable to the neuroleptics may contribute to sexual dysfunction as well. Anticholinergic blockade can result in

Table 9.7. Occurrence of Reported Sexual Side Effects.

Decreased Sexual desire: 33%
Erectile difficulty: 21.5%
Ejaculatory dysfunction: 18.7%
Orgasmic dysfunction: 19.3% of the women and 15.9% of the men
Amenorrhea: 21.7%
Galactorrhea: 5.3% of the women and 2.7% of the men
Gynecomastia: 3% of the women and 6% of the men

dryness of the mucous membranes, constipation, and urinary retention. Dopaminergic blockade in the basal ganglia can result in akinesia, stiffness, or akathisia. Sedation may occur via a number of different mechanisms.

"Atypical" antipsychotics: The introduction of clozapine to the U.S.A. in 1990 heralded the advent of a new class of antipsychotic agent. Clozapine differs from previous drugs in a number of ways: It is more effective in blocking the serotonin $5HT_2$ receptor than the dopamine D_2 receptors; it is effective for many treatment refractory patients; it is somewhat more efficacious than typical neuroleptics in the treatment of negative symptoms; it does not increase serum prolactin levels; it does not produce the movement disorders of the typical neuroleptics; and it does not appear to cause tardive dyskinesia. At times, the term "atypical" has been used to encompass some or all of these descriptors; however, more generally, it has been used to signify the lack of motor side effects. Clozapine was associated with a number of both bothersome (i.e., sedation, weight gain, drooling etc.), and potentially life-threatening (i.e., seizure, sudden death, agranulocytosis) side effects. This stimulated the search for agents that retained its more positive features, while, hopefully eliminating the side-effects.

Three other agents have subsequently been introduced. Risperidone was introduced in 1993, olanzapine in 1996, and quetiapine in 1997. All are associated with fewer motor side effects; their efficacy in treatment refractory patients is yet to be determined (Marder & Meibach, 1994; Tollefson et al., 1997). Risperidone is associated with a moderate increase in serum prolactin; olanzapine and quetiapine are associated with a mild transient increase in serum prolactin (Jibson & Tandon, 1996). Two other atypical agents (sertindole and ziprasidone) are in the process of being introduced; like risperidone, olanzapine, and quetiapine, they are effective in treating positive symptoms, appear more effective in treating negative symptoms, and are significantly less likely to cause extrapyramidal side-effects (Tollefson *et al.*, 1997; Tandon, Harrigan & Zorn, 1997). There are pharmacological differences between these various atypical agents as well, although the precise clinical implications of these differences are unclear (Jibson & Tandon, in press).

At this point little has been written about the propensity of these agents to cause sexual dysfunction. The impact of serotonergic-dopaminergic blockade versus dopaminergic blockade on sexual functioning is unknown. Some advantage for clozapine and some, but not all, of the other atypicals should be derived from the lack of effect on prolactin. However, clozapine produces pronounced anticholinergic and antihistaminic side effects, which can result in both direct and indirect effects on sexual functioning. The indirect effects on sexual functioning attributable to risperidone, olanzapine, and quetiapine are moderate. These agents can cause priapism, erectile difficulties, and ejaculatory dysfunction, although precise estimates of the frequency of the occurrence of these side effects are not known. There may be significant differences between various atypical agents with regard to propensity to cause sexual dysfunction (Jibson & Tandon, in press), and additional experience with these medications should inform us on this issue.

Management of sexual dysfunction secondary to antipsychotic agents: Gitlin (1994) has suggested a number of treatment strategies to decrease sexual dysfunction secondary to antipsychotic agents (see Table 9.8). The first step in management of sexual dysfunction secondary to an antipsychotic agent involves detection. Schizophrenic patients may be less likely than other patients to share this information, so it is vital that the physician question the patient specifically about sexual dysfunction. Dosage reduction may be beneficial given that sexual side effects, other than priapism, tend to be dose-related. If an anticholinergic agent is being used to manage the motor side effects of a conventional neuroleptic, substitution of amantadine may be helpful. In cases where the prolactin level is elevated, bromocriptine at dosages of 2.3 mg. two or three times a day may result in resolution of side effects. It should be noted that each of the two agents suggested above are dopamine agonists and may exacerbate psychosis. An alternative strategy in a case in which the offending agent is a conventional antipsychotic involves switching to an atypical agent, particularly risperidone or olanzapine.

Sildenafil citrate (Viagra) was released in 1998 as an oral therapy for erectile dysfunction. Following sexual stimulation, local release of nitric oxide in the corpus cavernosum activates guanylate cyclase, resulting in increased levels of cyclic guanosine monophosphate (cGMP). This leads to smooth muscle relaxation in the corpus cavernosum and inflow of blood resulting in erection. Sildenafil acts by inhibiting phosphodiesterase type 5 (PDE5), the enzyme responsible for the degradation of cGMH, enhancing the effect of nitric oxide and increasing the levels of cGMP in the corpus callosum. Sildenafil has been shown to be effective in a broad range of patients with erectile

Table 9.8. Management of Sexual Dysfunction Secondary to Antipsychotic Agents.

1. Question the patient specifically about sexual dysfunction.
2. Consider reducing the dosage of the antipsychotic agent.
3. Substitute amantadine if an anticholinergic agent is being used to manage extrapyramidal side effects.
4. If the prolactin level is elevated, add bromocriptine 2.3 mg. two or three times a day.
5. Switch from a conventional to an atypical agent.
6. Consider a trial of sildenafil citrate.
7. Treat priapism as a urologic emergency.

dysfunction, including those who take psychotropic medications. The recommended dosage is 50 mg. taken approximately one hour before sexual activity. Side effects include headache, flushing, dyspepsia, nasal congestion, urinary tract infection, abnormal vision, diarrhea, dizziness, and rash. However, these are described as mild to moderate in nature, and are generally transient. Given the above, sildenafil may prove to be a useful tool in sexual dysfunction associated with antipsychotic medications, and other psychotropic medications as well (Pfizer Inc, 1998).

Priapism should be considered a urologic emergency that requires immediate consultation with a urologist. Effective treatment (i.e., irrigation of the corpora cavernosa with either saline or metaraminol [an alpha agonist]) within the first 4–6 hours can reduce the need for surgery and the risk of permanent impotence (Thompson, Ware & Blashfield, 1990; Gitlin, 1994).

Antidepressants

Virtually all of the antidepressants can cause sexual dysfunction. The notable exceptions are bupropion and, perhaps, nefazodone. Inhibition of libido and/or delayed ejaculation/orgasm is most frequently cited, but erectile difficulties may also occur. The selective serotonin inhibitors and clomipramine are the most commonly associated with sexual dysfunction, followed by the monoamine oxidase inhibitors (MAOIs) and heterocyclic antidepressants. In 1987, Monteiro, Noshirvani, Marks & Lelliott reported reduced or total absence of orgasm/ejaculation in 95% of patients (23/24) prescribed clomipramine. Reports of fluoxetine-induced sexual dysfunction range from 8–75% (Patterson, 1993; Herman et al., 1990) whereas those for paroxetine and sertraline range from 15–40% (Physicians' Desk Reference [PDR], 1998). The incidence of sexual dysfunction associated with MAOIs is believed to be between 20% and 40%, while up to one-third of the patients treated with heterocyclics report sexual side effects (Harrison, et al., 1985; Harrison et al., 1986). The reported incidence parallels potentiation of serotonergic activity; serotonergic mechanisms are therefore felt to be the primary mechanism of antidepressant-induced sexual dysfunction, particularly ejaculatory or orgasmic dysfunction. The incidence of sexual dysfunction with venlafaxine is reported to be approximately 12% (predominantly ejaculatory dysfunction), with nefazodone one per cent (predominantly impotence), and with bupropion less than one per cent (PDR, 1998).

The range of antidepressant-induced sexual dysfunction is extensive. Although inhibited desire and retarded or absent ejaculation/orgasm are the most frequently reported, retarded or inhibited ejaculation, dyspareunia, menstrual irregularities or amenorrhea, breast pain or tenderness, galactorrhea, and gynecomastia have also been reported.

Indirect effects of the SSRIs include discomfort secondary to sleep disturbance, dizziness, nausea, anxiety, or restlessness. Sedation, weight gain, dizziness, and drying out of the mucous membranes may be associated with the TCAs and MAOIs.

The incidence of priapism linked to trazodone has been estimated at between 1 in 1,000 to 1 in 10,000. Unlike neuroleptic-induced priapism, priapism induced by trazodone tends to occur early in treatment and to be preceded by unusually prolonged nocturnal erections (Thompson *et al.*, 1990). As noted previously, priapism is a urologic emergency. It may require medical or surgical intervention and can result in permanent impotence if untreated.

Serotonergic antidepressants have also been linked to an unusual side effect involving spontaneous orgasm and yawning. In animals, the stretching-yawning/penile erection syndrome has been shown to occur in response to oxytocin injection or by the administration of dopaminergic agents that stimulate oxytocin activity. Drugs that block dopamine will not block the oxytocin-induced stretching-yawning/penile erection syndrome, but drugs that block oxytocin will prevent the syndrome from being triggered by oxytocin or dopaminergic drugs. Oxytocin-induced yawning and erection can also be blocked by the cholinergic antagonist atropine, indicating that oxytocin requires some cholinergic activity for its stimulation of this syndrome. The mechanism by which this response is precipitated in humans remains unclear.

Management of sexual dysfunction secondary to antidepressants: There are a number of general strategies that have been suggested for the management of antidepressant-induced sexual dysfunction (see Table 9.9). Dosage reduction is advocated, in hopes that the sexual side effects will resolve without loss of the antidepressant effect. This strategy may be most effective with medications that have a flat-dose response curve (i.e., the SSRIs). The effects of lowering the dosage of sertraline, paroxetine, or fluvoxamine should be apparent within a

Table 9.9. Management of Sexual Dysfunction Secondary to Antidepressants.

---

1. Consider reducing the dosage of the antidepressant agent.
2. Wait for the development of tolerance.
3. Switch to an antidepressant with less serotonergic activity.
4. Try one of the specific antidotes shown to have some efficacy for sexual dysfunction secondary to an antidepressant (i.e., cyproheptadine; yohimbine; bethanecol; a dopaminergic agent such as amantidine, magnesium pemoline, and dextroamphetamine; buspar; or nefazodone).
5. Consider a trial of sildenafil citrate.
6. Treat priapism as a urologic emergency.

---

week; it may require 4–6 weeks before the effect of dosage reduction is apparent for fluoxetine given its long half-life (Gitlin, 1995).

It has also been suggested that tolerance to the sexual side effects may develop. True tolerance is probably rare, but improvement in sexual functioning over a series of months has been reported (i.e., with sertraline and phenelzine). In addition to lowering the dose or awaiting the development of tolerance, a change in the dosing regimen may be helpful.

Switching to an agent that results in less serotonergic activity is the most frequent way in which antidepressant-induced sexual dysfunction is managed. Within the tricyclic class, switching from a more serotonergic agent or more anticholinergic agent (i.e., amitriptyline, imipramine) to a less serotonergic and less anticholinergic agent (i.e., desipramine, nortriptyline) is suggested. Bupropion and nefazodone are reasonable options to other classes of antidepressants given the low incidence of sexual side effects associated with each.

Bupropion is an antidepressant that exerts its antidepressant effect via dopamine uptake inhibition and weak norepinephrine uptake inhibition. Gardner and Johnston (1985) reported that drive and performance improved in 24 of 28 male patients switched from various antidepressants (mostly tricyclics) to bupropion. In a 1993 study by Walker *et al.*, 94% of patients switched from fluoxetine to bupropion due to sexual side effects reported partial or complete resolution of their fluoxetine-induced orgasmic difficulties and 81% reported improvement in libido from the level experienced while on fluoxetine. Bupropion has also been used in low dose (i.e., 75–150 mg./day) to reduce SSRI-induced sexual dysfunction.

Like trazodone, nefazodone is a serotonin reuptake inhibitor and $5HT_2$ receptor antagonist (Feiger *et al.*, 1996). However, it causes less blockade of the peripheral alpha$_1$ receptor than trazodone, and is therefore less likely to cause priapism. During investigatory clinical testing as an antidepressant, it was found to be less likely than other SSRIs to cause sexual dysfunction. This may be due to its preferential antagonism of the $5HT_2$ receptor. In fact, it was introduced in late 1994 as a possible alternative agent for patients who had benefited from an SSRI but experienced prohibitive sexual side effects. As mentioned for bupropion, nefazodone has also been used to reverse SSRI-induced sexual dysfunction (Reynolds, 1997).

If the more general strategies for the management of antidepressant-induced side effects are not successful or not tolerated, several specific agents have demonstrated benefit to certain patients. It should be emphasized that the literature relative to the these agents is sparse and consists largely of case reports or series. Cyproheptadine, yohimbine, bethanecol, and dopaminergic agents such as amantadine, magnesium pemoline, and dextroamphetamine are adjunctive agents employed to correct antidepressant-induced sexual dysfunction (Gitlin, 1995; Seagraves, 1993).

Cyproheptadine (Periactin) is an antihistamine with antiserotonergic properties, marketed for the treatment of allergic disorders. It has been shown to reverse anorgasmia caused by all classes of antidepressants, most probably secondary to its antiserotonergic effect. It may be administered on a scheduled or as needed basis in doses of between 2–16 mg. If it is taken on an as needed basis the dosage should be ingested one to two hours prior to initiation of sexual activity. The most common side effects associated with cyproheptadine are sedation and loss of antidepressant effect. Sedation may be severe enough to limit the usefulness of cyproheptadine as an antidote. Reversal of antidepressant effect may occur within hours to days of having started the cyproheptadine, and resolves quickly once the cyproheptadine is stopped.

In contrast to cyproheptadine, the presynaptic alpha$_2$ blocker, yohimbine, may have a broader scope of activity in the treatment of antidepressant-induced sexual dysfunction. It has been shown to reverse inhibition of libido, erectile dysfunction and anorgasmia induced by TCAs and serotonergic agents. Proposed mechanisms of action include a centrally mediated increase in libido and/or decreased venous outflow from the corpora cavernosa peripherally. Like cyproheptadine, yohimbine may be administered on a scheduled or as needed basis. When given on a scheduled basis, the typical dosage is 5.4 mg. three times a day; as needed doses range from 2.7–16.2 mg. Again, side effects may be limiting and include anxiety, nausea, insomnia, urinary urgency, and sweating. Theoretically, yohimbine might be associated with the risk of hypertensive reaction if used in combination with an MAOI.

Bethanecol (Urecholine), a cholinergic agonist, may reverse sexual dysfunction secondary to tricyclic antidepressants and monoamine oxidase inhibitors. Doses required are between 10–40 mg. as needed or 30–100 mg./day. Side effects include diarrhea, cramping, and excessive sweating.

Dopaminergic agents are another alternative for antidepressant-induced sexual side effects. Proposed mechanisms of action include the facilitation of dopamine activity centrally or reversal of the dopamine depleting action of the serotonergic medications. Amantadine, a dopamine agonist used in the treatment of parkinsonian symptoms and as an antiviral agent, has been reported to reverse fluoxetine-induced anorgasmia in days to weeks at a scheduled dose of 100–200 mg./day. Side effects are typically minimal. Both D-amphetamine and pemoline reversed decreased libido, erectile dysfunction, and anorgasmia in case reports. Again, side effects were minimal. However, the combination of a stimulant and an MAOI is potentially dangerous, resulting in a hypertensive reaction. The potential benefit of adding bupropion to a successful antidepressant trial complicated by sexual side effects was noted above.

Buspirone, a 5HT$_{1A}$ agonist indicated for the treatment of anxiety, has also been shown to be of benefit in the treatment of SSRI-induced inhibition of libido and anorgasmia. Dosage required is typically between 15–60 mg./day. As noted earlier, nefazodone has also been shown to reverse SSRI-induced anorgasmia at a dosage of 100–150 mg. taken an hour before a romantic episode.

Sildenafil citrate (Viagra) was released during year 1998 for the treatment of erectile dysfunction. Its indications include dysfunction secondary to psychotropic medication. It may prove to be a valuable tool in the treatment of erectile dysfunction secondary to antidepressant medication.

Mood Stabilizing Agents

Lithium: Lithium's effect on sexual functioning is poorly defined. Both desire disorders and erectile/orgasmic difficulties have been reported. However, the literature supporting these claims is sparse, comprised mostly of case reports or retrospective reviews (Blay, Ferraz, and Calil, 1980; Kristensen and Jorgensen, 1987; Page, Benaim, and Lappin, 1987; Ghadirian, Annable, and Belanger, 1992). A number of the reports are complicated/confounded by the concurrent use of other psychotropic medications. Lithium may be associated with sexual dysfunction indirectly via its propensity to induce weight gain, polyuria, loss of spontaneity, etc.

Patient complaints of altered sexual functioning should be evaluated in the context of the disorder itself, recognizing that hypersexuality is frequently a symptom of an untreated bipolar disorder. Hypersexuality due to mania or hypomania resolves with adequate treatment of the underlying disorder. However, physicians should not fail to respond to patient concerns regarding sexual functioning based on the assumption that the patient is simply pining for the hypomanic or manic state. When a patient taking lithium and other psychotropics complains of sexual side effects, elimination of concurrent psychotropic medications (when possible) may resolve the difficulties. If this is not feasible, a trial of valproate may be indicated.

Anticonvulsants: Valproate, FDA approved for the treatment of bipolar disorder in 1995, appears to be relatively free of direct sexual side effects. Unlike other anticonvulsants, it does not inhibit the adrenal androgens or increase prolactin levels. Like lithium, its major effect on sexual function may be indirect and related to sedation, nausea, weight gain, etc.

Carbamazepine, via its stimulation of liver enzymes, results in decreased circulating levels of the androgens. Prolactin levels are also increased. Indirect effects on sexual functioning include sedation, weight gain, dizziness, and fatigue. Additional concerns as to bone marrow suppression and agranulocytosis or aplastic anemia have resulted in its being relegated to a second-line choice for the treatment of bipolar disorder, apart from its effect on sexual functioning. Finally, if used in conjunction with an oral contraceptive agent, an increase in dosage of the oral contraceptive agent may be necessary for continued contraceptive efficacy.

Antianxiety Agents

Benzodiazepines: A number of different agents are available for the treatment of anxiety. The benzodiazepines are probably the most widely used, despite ever-present concerns about the development of tolerance and withdrawal. The notion that benzodiazepines affect sexual functioning positively secondary to anxiety reduction is attractive, but misguided. In fact, benzodiazepines cause or aggravate sexual dysfunction in both men and women. Benzodiazepines stimulate endogenous benzodiazepine receptors and facilitate GABA transmission in the limbic area, lessening attention and emotional reactivity (Crenshaw and Goldberg, 1996). Desire is reduced, particularly when high doses are involved, and dysfunction related to ejaculation and orgasm has also been reported most likely resulting from decreases in alpha$_1$ adrenergic activity, LHRH, and testosterone.

Indirect side effects can also result in sexual dysfunction. Sedation and cognitive deficits can lead to decreased desire and enjoyment. Disinhibition can result in sexual involvement that might not otherwise occur. Aggressive and hostile reactions may lead to unfortunate consequences. These effects can be exacerbated with the concurrent use of alcohol.

Buspirone: Buspirone is an attractive alternative to a benzodiazepine. Buspirone is a 5HT1 agonist marketed for the treatment of generalized anxiety. No direct sexual side effects have been reported for buspirone. In fact, as noted in the section on antidepressant medications, it has been used to treat antidepressant-induced sexual dysfunction with some success. In addition, it does not cause sedation or cognitive impairment, and does not potentiate the effect of alcohol. Some discomfort may occur as a result of headache, nausea, or tremor, but these effects may dissipate with time. Unfortunately, buspirone is not effective for panic disorder and may be less effective in patients previously exposed to benzodiazepines.

Beta-blockers: Beta-blockers have classically been used in the treatment of hypertension and migraine headaches. They have also been shown to be of benefit in treating performance anxiety or stage fright. The beta-blockers decrease the peripheral manifestations of anxiety (i.e., tremulousness, sweating, tachycardia) resulting in less somatic awareness of discomfort. However, these agents negatively affect sexual functioning by their affect on beta-adrenergic activity and, indirectly, by increasing serotonin levels. This results in impairment of desire and erection. Studies have indicated that up to 23% of men treated with propranolol become impotent, although the percentages are suspect given that other antihypertensive medications were being administered concurrently (Hogan, Wallin and Baer, 1980). Side-effects such as orthostatic hypotension, fatigue, etc., may also affect sexual functioning. The association between beta-blockers and depression also needs to be considered when using a beta blocker.

Management of sexual dysfunction secondary to antianxiety agents: As with each of the classes of medication reviewed thus far, several general measures can be suggested for management of the sexual side effects associated with the anxiolytics (see Table 9.10). Given that sexual side effects appear to be more common with higher doses of a benzodiazepine, dosage reduction is advocated as a first step when possible. Switching to buspirone may be a reasonable option when treating generalized anxiety disorder. Cognitive behavioral therapy, which has demonstrated equal efficacy to medication in panic disorder, may be suggested when sexual dysfunction complicates treatment with alprazolam or clonazepam. The use of antidepressant medications (i.e., SSRIs, TCAs, or MAOIs), while having clearly demonstrated broad efficacy across the spectrum of anxiety disorders, may not offer any benefit over the anxiolytic medications in terms of sexual dysfunction given their proclivity to cause sexual dysfunction.

Table 9.10. Management of Sexual Dysfunction Secondary to Antianxiety Agents.

1. Consider reducing the dosage of the antianxiety agent.
2. Switch to buspar when treating a generalized anxiety disorder.
3. Consider CBT as an alternative treatment for panic disorder.

CONCLUSION

Sexual activity is an integral aspect of human life. While this is obvious, its importance in the treatment of our patients is often overlooked. Sexual dysfunction is frequently experienced by patients with various psychiatric disorders; it can also be induced by all classes of psychotropic medication. Distinguishing illness-associated sexual dysfunction from that induced by medications can be extremely difficult. In the preceding pages, we have sought to acquaint the reader with sexual side effects associated with each class of psychotropic medication. Both general, and, when available, more specific recommendations for management have been suggested. Application of this information should serve to minimize the patient's discomfort and improve quality of life, hopefully resulting in enhanced compliance and better treatment outcomes.

REFERENCES

Blay, S.L., Ferraz, M.P.T. & Calil, H.M. (1982). Lithium-induced male sexual impairment: Two case reports. *Journal of Clinical Psychiatry* 43:497–498.

Crenshaw, T.L. & Goldberg, J.P. (1996). *Sexual pharmacology: Drugs that affect sexual functioning.* New York, London: W.W. Norton & Company.

DeLeo, D. & Magni, G. (1983). Sexual side-effects of antidepressant drugs. *Psychosomatics* 24:1076–1082.

Feiger, A., Kiev, A., Shrivastava, R.K., Wisselink, P.G. & Wilcox, C.S. (1996). Nefazodone versus sertraline in outpatients with major depression: Focus on efficacy, tolerability, and effects on sexual function and satisfaction. *Journal of Clinical Psychiatry* 57:(Suppl 2), 53–62.

Finn, S.E., Bailey, J.M., Schultz, R.T. & Faber, R. (1990). Subjective utility ratings of neuroleptics in treating schizophrenia. *Psychological Medicine,* 20:843–848.

Gardner, E.A. & Johnston, J.A. (1985). Bupropion — an antidepressant without sexual pathophysiological action. *Journal of Clinical Psychopharmacology* 5:24–29.

Gitlin, M.J. (1995). Effects of depression and antidepressants on sexual functioning. *Bulletin of the Menninger Clinic* 59: 232–248.

Gitlin, M.J. (1994). Psychotropic medications and their effects on sexual function: Diagnosis, biology, and treatment approaches. *Journal of Clinical Psychiatry* 55:406–413.

Ghadirian, A.M., Annable, L. & Belanger, M.C. (1992). Lithium, benzodiazepines, and sexual function in bipolar patients. *American Journal of Psychiatry* 149:801–805.

Harrison, W.M., Rabkin, J.G., Ehrhardt, A.A., Stewart, J.W., McGrath, P.J., Ross, D. & Quitkin, F.M. (1986). Effects of antidepressant medication on sexual function: a controlled study. *Journal of Clinical Psychopharmacology* 6:144–149.

Harrison, W.M., Stewart, J., Ehrhardt, A.A., Rabkin, J., McGrath, P., Liebowitz, M. & Quitkin, F.M. (1985). A controlled study of the effects of antidepressants on sexual function. *Psychopharmacology Bulletin* 21:85–88.

Hogan, J.H., Wallin, J.D. & Baer, R.M. (1980). Antihypertensive therapy and male sexual dysfunction. *Psychosomatics* 21:234–237.

Herman, J.B., Brotman, A.W., Pollack, M.H., Falk, W.E., Biederman, J. & Rosenbaum, J.F. (1990). Fluoxetine-induced sexual dysfunction. *Journal of Clinical Psychiatry* 51:25–27.

Jibson, M.D. & Tandon, R. (1996). A summary of research findings on the new antipsychotic drugs. *Directions in Psychiatry* 16:i–viii.

Jibson, M.D. & Tandon, R. (In Press). Atypical antipsychotics: How do they compare. *Journal of Psychiatric Research,* In Press.

Kristensen, E. & Jorgensen, P. (1987). Sexual function in lithium-treated manic-depressive patients. *Pharmacopsychiatry* 20:165–167.

Lingjaerde, O., Ahlfors, U.G., Bech, P., Dencker, S.J. & Elgen, K. (1987). The UKU side-effect rating scale: A new comprehensive rating scale for psychotropic drugs and a cross-sectional study of side effects in neuroleptic-treated patients. *Acta Psychiatrica Scandinavia* 76:(Suppl. 334) 1–99.

Marder, S.R. & Meibach, R.C. (1994). Risperidone in the treatment of schizophrenia. *American Journal of Psychiatry* 151:825–835.

Monteiro, W.O., Noshirvani, H.F., Marks, I.M. & Lelliott, P.T. (1987). Anorgasmia from clomipramine in obsessive-compulsive disorder: A controlled trial. *British Journal of Psychiatry* 151:1007–112.

Page, C., Benaim, S. & Lappin, F. (1987). A long-term retrospective follow-up study of patients treated with prophylactic lithium carbonate. *British Journal of Psychiatry* 150:175–179.

Patterson, W.M. (1993). Fluoxetine-induced sexual dysfunction. *Journal of Clinical Psychiatry* (letter to the editor) 54: 71.

Montvale, N.J. (1998). *Physicians' Desk Reference* (51st ed.). Medical Economics Company, Inc.

Reynolds, R.D. (1997). Sertraline-induced anorgasmia treated with intermittent nefazodone. *Journal of Clinical Psychiatry* (letter to the editor), 58: 89.

Schiavi, R.C. & Schreiner-Engel, P. (1980). Physiologic aspects of sexual function and dysfunction. *Psychiatric Clinics of North America* 3:81–95.

Seagraves, R.T. (1993). Treatment-emergent sexual dysfunction in affective disorder: A review and management strategies. *Journal of Clinical Psychiatry Monograph* 11:57–60.

Seagraves, R.T. (1989). Effects of psychotropic drugs on human erection and ejaculation. *Archives of General Psychiatry* 46:275–284.

Tandon, R., Harrigan, E. & Zorn, S.H. (1997). Ziprasidone: A novel antipsychotic with unique pharmacology and therapeutic potential. *Journal of Serotonin Research* 4:159–177.

Thompson, J.W., Ware, M.R. & Blashfield, R.K. (1990). Psychotropic medication and priapism: A comprehensive review. *Journal of Clinical Psychiatry* 51:430–433.

Tollefson, G.D., Beasley, C.M., Tran, P.V., Street, J.S., Krueger, J.A., Tamura, R.N., Graffeo, K.A. & Thieme, M.E. (1997). Olanzapine versus haloperidol in the treatment of schizophrenia and schizoaffective and schizophreniform disorders: Results of an international collaborative trial. *American Journal of Psychiatry* 154: 457–465.

Vander, A.J, Sherman, J.H. & Luciano, D.S. (1994). *Human Physiology: The mechanisms of body function.* (6th ed.). United States of America: McGraw-Hill, Inc.

Viagra (sildenafil citrate). Full prescribing information. (1998). Pfizer, Inc.

Walker, P.W., Cole, J.O., Gardner, E.A., Hughes, A.R., Johnston, J.A., Batey, S.R. & Lineberry, C.G. (1993). Improvement in fluoxetine-associated sexual dysfunction in patients switched to bupropion. *Journal of Clinical Psychiatry* 54:459–465.

10

Pharmacologic Management of Abnormal Sexual Behavior

SUSAN L. McELROY, CESAR A. SOUTULLO and PAUL E. KECK, JR.

Abnormal sexual behavior is an underrecognized problem among persons with mental illness. Such behavior may be broadly classified into three main categories: sexual hypofunction or dysfunction; sexual hyperfunction or excessive "normal" or conventional sexual behavior; and "deviant" or unconventional sexual behavior. Sexual hyperfunction and deviant sexual behavior may be further subdivided into aggressive and nonaggressive forms.

Each of these categories of abnormal sexual behavior has multiple etiologies, and some forms of such behavior may respond to treatment with pharmacologic agents. Thus, for any patient presenting with abnormal sexual behavior, the etiology, or etiologies, of that behavior should be determined. The etiology of the abnormal sexual behavior will help clarify whether pharmacologic treatment might be helpful, and what that treatment should entail.

In this chapter, disorders associated with abnormal sexual behavior are first reviewed. Then, pharmacologic agents with effects on sexual behavior are discussed. Suggested recommendations for the evaluation and pharmacologic management of abnormal sexual behavior are then presented.

I. Disorders Associated with Abnormal Sexual Behavior

Sexual dysfunction: In DSM-IV, sexual dysfunctions are defined as disturbances in the processes that characterize the sexual response cycle (which is divided into desire, excitement, orgasm, and resolution) that cause marked distress or interpersonal difficulty (American Psychiatric Association, 1994). Specific types of sexual dysfunctions included in DSM-IV are: sexual desire disorders (i.e., hypoactive sexual desire disorder and sexual aversion disorder); sexual arousal disorders (i.e., female sexual arousal disorder and male erectile disorder [also called impotence and defined as the inability to maintain an erection sufficient for intercourse]); orgasmic disorders (i.e., female and male orgasmic disorders, premature ejaculation); sexual pain disorder (i.e., dyspareunia and vaginismus); sexual dysfunction due to a general medical condition; substance induced-sexual dysfunction; and sexual dysfunction not otherwise specified (NOS).

Surprisingly little is known about the psychosexual dysfunctions in persons with mental illness or, conversely, about the psychopathology of persons with sexual dysfunctions. However, preliminary data suggest that some of these disorders may be responsive to pharmacologic interventions. For example, clinical experience suggests that anxiolytic agents (e.g., alprazolam) in low-to-moderate doses may reduce anxiety and panic associated with sexual aversion disorder without causing sedation or interfering with sexual functioning (Kaplan, 1995). Double blind, placebo-controlled trials have shown that the serotonin reuptake inhibitors clomipramine (Girgis et al., 1982; Goodman, 1980) and paroxetine (Waldinger et al., 1994) are effective in premature ejaculation. Reduced libido in hypogonadal men and postmenopausal women may respond to androgenic agents (Pope & Katz, in press). Male erectile dysfunction of organic and/or psychogenic origin has been shown to respond to oral administration of the α 2-adrenoreceptor antagonist yohimbine (Reid et al., 1987; Riley et al., 1989; Susset et al., 1989), the opiate antagonist naltrexone (Fabbri et al., 1989), the dopamine receptor antagonists apomorphine and bromocriptine (Cooper, 1977; Lal et al., 1989; Gregoire, 1992), and most recently, the GMP-specific phosphodiesterase inhibitor sildenafil (Boolell et al., 1996a & b; Goldstein et al., 1998; Terrett et al., 1996). Male erectile dysfunction may also respond to self-administered injections of vasoactive drugs, such as papaverine plus phentolamine and prostaglandin E1, into the corpora cavernosa of the penis (Gregoire, 1992; Schiavi, 1995).

Paraphilias and nonparaphilic sexual addictions: In DSM-IV, paraphilias are defined as sexual disorders characterized by recurrent, intense, sexually arousing fantasies, sexual urges, or sexual behaviors generally involving nonhuman objects, the suffering or humiliation of oneself or one's partner, or children or other nonconsenting persons (American Psychiatric Association, 1994).

DSM-IV further specifies that the sexual fantasies, urges, or behaviors occur over a period of at least six months and cause clinically significant distress or impairment in functioning. Paraphilias listed in DSM-IV are exhibitionism (the exposure of one's genitals), fetishism (the use of nonliving objects), frotteurism (the touching and rubbing against a nonconsenting person), pedophilia (sexual fantasies or activity involving a prepubescent child), sexual masochism (deriving sexual excitement from the act of being humiliated), sexual sadism (deriving sexual excitement from the psychological or physical suffering of others), transvestic fetishism (cross-dressing), voyeurism (observing unsuspecting strangers who are naked, disrobing, or engaging in sexual activity) and paraphilias not otherwise specified (NOS). Examples of the NOS category include telephone scatologia (obscene phone calls), necrophilia (corpses), partialism (body parts), zoophilias (animals), coprophilia (feces), klismaphilia (enemas), urophilia (urine), and autoerotic asphyxiation (strangulation while masturbating). Of note, persons with paraphilias (at least those who commit sexual crimes) tend to have multiple paraphilias (Abel *et al.*, 1988; Bradford *et al.*, 1992).

Nonparaphilic sexual addictions (NPSAs), also called compulsive sexual behaviors or sexual compulsions, are not included in DSM-IV as formal mental disorders, but are possible examples of sexual disorders NOS. They have been defined as repetitive sexual acts and intrusive sexual thoughts involving "normal,"conventional, or nondeviant sexual behaviors which a person feels compelled or driven to perform, which may or may not cause subjective distress (Anthony & Hollander, 1993; Black *et al.*, 1997; Coleman, 1987; Kafka, 1991a, 1994a, 1995; Kafka & Prentky, 1992a). Examples include compulsive or excessive masturbation, compulsive or protracted promiscuity, telephone sex, dependence on pornography or sexual "accessories" to achieve or maintain sexual arousal, or severe incompatibility between partners because of differing degrees of sexual desire. As with persons with paraphilias, persons with NPSAs tend to have multiple sexual addictions. Although paraphilias and NPSAs are distinguished from each other by the abnormality or "deviance" of the sexual fantasies or behaviors, there is considerable overlap between these two conditions. Indeed, many persons with paraphilias also have NPSAs (Kafka, 1994a; Kafka & Prentky, 1992a).

Preliminary phenomenologic, comorbidity, and treatment response data suggest that paraphilias and NPSAs are bona-fide mental illnesses that are related to other major psychiatric disorders, especially mood, obsessive-compulsive, impulse control, and substance use disorders (Black *et al.*, 1997; Hollander, 1993; Hollander & Wong, 1995; Kafka, 1994a, 1995; McElroy *et al.*, 1993, 1996). Regarding phenomenologic similarities, paraphilic and NPSA impulses and behaviors are often experienced as compulsive, uncontrollable, or irresistible, as are the obsessions and compulsions of obsessive-compulsive disorder (OCD), the impulses and behaviors of impulse control disorders (ICDs), and the cravings and alcohol and drug use of substance use disorders (Perilstein *et al.*, 1991; Pearson, 1990; Zohar *et al.*, 1994). Indeed, DSM-IV states that paraphilias are forms of impulse control disorders. Moreover, paraphilic impulses may be associated with anxiety, tension, or depressed mood similar to that of major depression, and paraphilic behaviors may be associated with euphoria similar to that of hypomania (Croughan *et al.*, 1981).

Comorbidity studies indicate that men with paraphilias have elevated rates of mood, obsessive-compulsive, impulse control, and substance use disorders. For example, in an interview of 70 male members of cross dressing clubs, Croughan *et al.* (1981) reported that 30% of the subjects met definite or probable Feighner *et al.* (1972) criteria for a lifetime diagnosis of unipolar depression, six percent for obsessional neurosis, 24% for alcoholism, and 22% for drug use. Of 15 men with DSM-III-R paraphilias evaluated by Kruesi *et al.* (1992), nine (60%) met lifetime RDC criteria for a mood disorder, six (40%) for an anxiety disorder, and eight (53%) for a substance use disorder. Of 20 men with NPSAs recruited by newspaper advertisement for the evaluation and treatment of "sexual addictions/compulsions," 10 of whom had a NPSA and no paraphilia and 10 of whom had a NPSA and at least one DSM-III-R paraphilia, 19 (95%) met DSM-III-R criteria for a history of dysthymia and 11 (55%) met criteria for current major depression (Kafka & Prentzky, 1992b). Of 10 patients with paraphilias and/or NPSAs evaluated by Stein *et al.*(1992), seven (70%) had comorbid OCD. Of 60 consecutive male outpatients seeking treatment for a paraphilia (N=26) or a NPSA (N=34) evaluated by Kafka and Prentky (1994), 47% displayed a lifetime history of a substance use disorder. Of 22 adolescent males who admitted to sexually molesting a child at least once evaluated by our group, all of whom met DSM-IV criteria for at least one paraphilia, 18 (82%) met lifetime criteria for a mood disorder, six (27%) for OCD, 12 (55%) for an ICD, and 11 (50%) for a substance use disorder (Galli *et al.*, 1999). More recently, of 36 men with compulsive sexual behaviors recruited by newspaper advertisement (seven [19%] whose "main impulsive sexual behavior" was paraphilic) evaluated by Black *et al.*, (1997), 14 (39%) reported a lifetime history of major depression or dysthymia, 15 (42%) a history of phobic disorder, and 23 (64%) a history of substance use disorder.

Preliminary treatment response data suggest that paraphilias and NPSAs may respond to medications effective in mood, obsessive-compulsive, and impulse control disorders, including antidepressants (e.g., tricyclics and serotonin reuptake inhibitors [SRIs]) (Federoff, 1993; Kafka, 1991a & b, 1994a & b, 1995; Kafka & Prentky, 1992b; Greenberg & Bradford, 1997) and mood stabilizers (e.g., lithium) (Cesnik & Coleman, 1989; Kafka 1991a; Ward, 1975). For example, in an open-label, 12-week study of fluoxetine (mean dose = 39 mg) in 20 men with NPSA's (either alone [N=10] or with at least one paraphilia),

Kafka and Prentzky (1992b) reported significant reductions in excessive and deviant sexual symptoms after four weeks of treatment without adverse effects on conventional sexual behavior. In a controlled comparison of clomipramine and desipramine in 15 men with paraphilias, both drugs were equally superior to a single-blind, two week baseline treatment period with placebo in the eight men who completed the trial (Kruesi et al., 1992). By contrast, a recent controlled case study of a male patient with exhibitionism treated with fluvoxamine, desipramine, and placebo in a crossover design suggested that some paraphilic patients may respond preferentially to SRIs (Zohar et al., 1994). In this patient, fluvoxamine eliminated "abnormal" sexual impulses and behavior without affecting "normal" sexual desire, whereas desipramine and placebo were both associated with relapse.

Based on these data, our group and others have hypothesized that the paraphilias and NPSAs belong to a family of disorders related to OCD and the ICDs, which we have termed the compulsive-impulsive spectrum disorders (Anthony & Hollander, 1993; Hollander, 1993; McElroy et al., 1993, 1996; Pearson, 1990). Disorders in this family are characterized by the compulsive and/or impulsive performance of senseless or harmful behaviors or, more broadly, a core disturbance in compulsivity and/or impulsivity. This family of disorders has been hypothesized to include OCD, intermittent explosive disorder, kleptomania, pathological gambling, pyromania, trichotillomania, eating disorders, tic disorders, and some forms of substance abuse, among others. In light of mounting evidence indicating that OCD, the ICDs, and most other forms of compulsive-impulsive spectrum disorders are related to mood disorder, our group has also hypothesized that the compulsive-impulsive spectrum disorders (including the paraphilias) may belong to the larger family of affective spectrum disorder. Affective spectrum disorder is a hypothesized family of disorders – including depressive disorders, bipolar disorders, OCD, most other anxiety disorders, bulimia and anorexia nervosa, and attention deficit hyperactivity disorder among others – that share high comorbidity with mood disorder, high familial rates of mood disorder, and response to thymoleptic agents (i.e., antidepressants and/or mood stabilizers), and thus, possibly a common pathophysiologic abnormality with mood disorder (McElroy et al., 1993, 1996).

However, there are important differences between paraphilias, NPSAs, and ICDs on the one hand, and OCD on the other. First, paraphilias, NPSAs, and certain ICDs (e.g., intermittent explosive disorder, pathological gambling, pyromania) are more common in men, whereas OCD is equally common in both sexes. Second, although systematic phenomenologic comparison studies have not yet been conducted, paraphilic, NPSA, and ICD symptoms are probably more often associated with pleasurable feelings (especially sexual pleasure for paraphilias and NPSAs) and are more likely to be enacted, and thus, are more likely to be impulsive and ego-syntonic than are OCD symptoms. Paraphilias, NPSAs, and ICDs may also be associated with higher rates of comorbid conditions with impulsive features than is OCD, such as bipolar disorder, substance use disorders, criminal behavior, and borderline and antisocial personality disorders (McElroy *et al.*, 1996). For example, of the 22 adolescent male sex offenders evaluated by our group, all of whom had at least one paraphilia, 12 (54%) had bipolar disorder and 11 (50%) had a substance use disorder. Similarly, of the 15 men with paraphilias evaluated by Kruesi *et al.* (1992), eight (53%) had substance abuse and four (27%) had antisocial personality disorder. Finally, individuals with paraphilias and other ICDs have been reported to respond to thymoleptic agents other than SRIs, including non-SRI antidepressants and lithium (Cesnik & Coleman, 1989; Kruesi *et al.*, 1992; Ward, 1975). Indeed, as noted earlier, in one of the two controlled comparison trials conducted to date in paraphilias, clomipramine and desipramine were equally effective in suppressing paraphilic symptoms in the eight men who completed the study (Kruesi *et al.*, 1992).

To explain the similarities and differences among the disorders in the compulsive-impulsive spectrum disorder family, we have hypothesized that compulsivity and impulsivity might each be related to mood dysregulation, with depression (or unipolarity) sharing features with compulsivity, mania (or bipolarity) sharing features with impulsivity, and mixed affective states similar to mixtures of compulsivity and impulsivity (McElroy *et al.*, 1996). Specifically, compulsivity and depression are each characterized by inhibited or ruminative thinking and behavior, maintenance of insight or ego-dystonicity, and less marked fluctuations in mood state, with dysphoria typically alternating with relief rather than with euphoria or pleasurable feelings. Conversely, impulsivity and mania (or bipolarity) are each characterized by disinhibited or facilitated thinking and behavior, poor insight or ego-syntonicity, and more marked changes in mood state between dysphoric and pleasurable affects.

We have further hypothesized that the compulsive-impulsive spectrum disorders might be arranged along an axis (or related axes) of compulsivity-unipolarity versus impulsivity/bipolarity, where disorders characterized by maximum compulsivity and unipolarity (e.g., OCD with a comorbid depressive disorder) are at one end of this axis, and those with maximum impulsivity and bipolarity (e.g., a paraphilia with a comorbid bipolar disorder) are at the other (see Figure 10.1). Various mixed compulsive-impulsive forms would be situated in between, such as OCD with poor insight or impulsive features, ICDs with good insight or compulsive features, and the co-occurrence of OCD and an ICD in the same individual. Indeed, the sexual disorders might span such a dimension from compulsivity to impulsivity, with OCD with sexual obsessions at the compulsive extreme, paraphilias at the impulsive extreme, and the NPSAs and various mixed forms

High Compulsivity/ Unipolarity	Mixed Compulsive- Impulsive and/or Affective States	High Impulsivity / Bipolarity
OCD with Sexual Obsessions/ Depressive Disorders	NPSAs, Compulsive Paraphilias / Bipolar II Disorder	Paraphilias/ Bipolar I Disorder
Serotenergic Agents (SRIs) Other Antidepressants	Combinations of Agents	Mood Stabilizers Dopamine Antagonists Antiandrogen Agents
Fluoxetine, Sertraline Bupropion	SRI + Mood Stabilizer SRI + Antiandrogen Mood Stabilizer + Antiandrogen	Lithium Valproate Antipsychotics MPA

Figure 10.1. Hypothesized relationship among impulsivity, compulsivity, affective dysregulation, abnormal sexual behaviour, and pharmacological treatment response.

(e.g., OCD and a paraphilia occurring in the same individual or a paraphilia with compulsive features) situated in between (see Figure 10.1). Tentative support for such a dimension comes from preliminary data suggesting that more impulsive disorders (i.e., paraphilias, ICDs) may be associated with higher rates of bipolar relative to depressive disorders as compared to more compulsive disorders (i.e., OCD), and by possible differences in thymoleptic responsiveness of various compulsive-impulsive spectrum disorders, with more compulsive forms responding preferentially to SRIs, and more impulsive forms responding to a broader range of thymoleptics (e.g., to mood stabilizers and/or non-SRI antidepressants as well as to or instead of SRIs) (McElroy et al., 1996).

Mood disorders: Mood disorders are often accompanied by changes in sexual drive, function, and behavior. For example, the manic and mixed phases of bipolar disorder are often accompanied by increased libido and hypersexual behavior. In a review of seven studies of activity and behavior symptoms during mania in 224 patients with bipolar disorder, Goodwin & Jamison (1990) reported that 57% (range 27%–80%) displayed hypersexuality. Of note, hypersexuality in mania may reflect psychosis. In a study examining the relationship between psychotic features and other manic symptoms, Young et al. (1983) found that psychotic patients with mania were significantly more likely than nonpsychotic patients to have increased sexual interest, along with elevated mood, increased psychomotor activity and energy, and subjective sleep-disturbance.

Conversely, the depressive episodes of depressive and bipolar disorders are often associated with reduced libido, sexual dysfunction, and hyposexual behavior. Less frequently, they may be associated with hypersexual behavior, particularly if there is a comorbid NPSA or paraphilia. Thus, it is important that the presence of a mood disorder (both bipolar and depressive) be considered in the differential diagnosis of any patient presenting with a change in their sexual drive, function, or behavior.

Other axis I disorders: Other Axis I disorders may be characterized by abnormal sexual ideation and/or behavior. Persons with obsessive-compulsive disorder (OCD) may have sexual obsessions that involve sexual thoughts or imagery (e.g., a recurrent pornographic image) (Stein et al., 1992). Of note, it is sometimes difficult to distinguish the sexual impulses of paraphilias and NPSAs from the sexual obsessions of OCD, particularly when the former are ego dystonic and not enacted (Hollander & Wong, 1995). Persons with phobic disorders or post traumatic stress disorder may have various sexual phobias. Persons with psychotic disorders, especially those in the manic or mixed phase of schizoaffective disorder, bipolar type, or those with the erotomanic subtype of delusional disorder, may present with hypersexual behavior that may be delusional in etiology.

Finally, persons with Tourette's disorder may have sexual obsessions, corprolalia, and/or impulsive sexual behaviors.

Axis II disorders and psychopathy: Borderline and antisocial personality disorders and psychopathy all are often characterized by excessive, promiscuous, and/or self-destructive sexual behaviors that have a high risk for harmful consequences. For example, DSM-IV lists "impulsivity in sex" that is "potentially self-damaging" as a diagnostic criteria for borderline personality disorder (American Psychiatric Association, 1994), and persons with antisocial personality disorder or psychopathy may be irresponsible, exploitative, and even sadistic in their sexual relationships (Meloy, 1997). Indeed, although not extensively studied, preliminary data suggest that persons with borderline and antisocial personality disorders may have elevated rates of paraphilias and other disturbances of sexual behavior (Virkkunen, 1976). For example, in a study of the sexual histories of 80 patients who met DSM-III criteria (American Psychiatric Association, 1980) for borderline personality disorder, Zubenko et al. (1987) reported that 9 (11%) had paraphilias.

Borderline or antisocial personality disorder and/or psychopathy must therefore be considered in the differential diagnosis of any patient exhibiting excessive "normal" or any degree of deviant sexual behavior, particularly if the behavior is impulsive, self-destructive, or exploitative. However, the pharmacologic treatment of abnormal sexual behavior due to personality disorders or psychopathy has not been studied, and at present, no known medical treatment for it exists. Current pharmacologic treatment of such sexual behavior, therefore, usually depends on targeting comorbid Axis I disorders or symptoms (e.g., SRIs or antiandrogen agents for comorbid paraphilias or NPSAs, or thymoleptics for comorbid affective symptoms or mood disorders).

Medical disorders: Numerous medical disorders may cause sexual dysfunction or other abnormal sexual behavior. These disorders include neurologic, endocrinologic, metabolic, and infectious illnesses, as well as reactions to medications or toxins. Examples include brain damage (especially involving the frontal and/or temporal lobes), dementia (including that due to Huntington's disease), epilepsy, encephalitis, diabetes, and various types of substance use disorders (Bell & Trethowan, 1961; Carner et al., 1993; Carrier et al., 1993; Fedoroff et al., 1994; Goldberg & Buongiorno, 1982–83; Hucker et al., 1988; O'Donohue & Geer, 1993). These etiologies should be considered in any patient with a primary mental disorder who develops abnormal sexual behavior, even if the behavior could be attributed to the mental disorder.

The relationship of sexual behavior to mental illness and also the lack thereof is described in detail elsewhere in this book (see Chapters 1,2,6).

II. Pharmacologic Agents that Affect Sexual Behavior

Agents that enhance sexual function: It is well documented that androgenic steroids enhance sexual drive in men and women (Pope & Katz, in press). Indeed, androgenic agents have been shown to restore sexual drive and ejaculatory function in hypogonadal men (O'Carroll & Bancroft, 1984; O'Carroll et al., 1985; Rabkin & Wagner, 1995) and to increase libido in post menopausal women (Sands & Shedd, 1995; Sherwin & Gelfand, 1985). Mounting research further indicates that these agents have antidepressant properties, may increase irritability and aggressivity, and may even induce manic-like symptoms in vulnerable persons, especially at high doses (Pope & Katz, in press).

Controlled studies have shown the α_2 antagonist yohimbine (Morales et al., 1987; Nelson, 1988; Reid et al., 1987; Riley et al., 1989; Susset et al., 1989) and, more recently, the GMP – specific phosphodiesterase inhibitor sildenafil (Boolell et al., 1996a & b; Goldstein et al., 1998; Terrett et al., 1996) to be effective in male erectile dysfunction of psychogenic and/or organic etiology. A recent study by Mann et al. (1996), however, suggested that yohimbine was more effective in men with nonorganic than organic erectile dysfunction. Male erectile dysfunction has also been shown in isolated studies to respond to the dopamine receptor agonist bromocriptine (Lal et al., 1989) and the opioid antagonist naltrexone (Fabbri et al., 1989). In addition, numerous agents have been reported to be effective in case reports and small open trials to reverse sexual dysfunction associated with various psychotropic agents, especially antidepressants and antipsychotics. These agents include yohimbine, the cholinergic agent bethanecol, dopamine agonists such as amantadine and psychostimulants, norepinephrine agonists such as bupropion, and serotonin antagonists such as cyproheptadine, buspirone, and granisetron (Gitlin, 1994; Nelson et al., 1997). However, it is important to note that none of the latter agents has yet been studied in the treatment of psychotropic-induced sexual dysfunction in controlled trials.

Antipsychotic agents: Antipsychotic agents affect sexual behavior in several ways (also see Millner, Chapter 9). First, they are associated with a wide range of types of sexual dysfunction, including reduced libido, erectile dysfunction, and retrograde ejaculation. These effects are thought to be due to a variety of mechanisms of action, including dopamine and adrenergic receptor blockade, and prolactin elevation (Kane & Lieberman, 1992; Seagraves, 1989). Second, these agents may effectively reduce hypersexuality and other abnormal sexual behavior due to mania or psychosis. Third, antipsychotics have been reported in isolated case reports (Maletzky, 1991) and open series (Bartholomew, 1968) to decrease sexual arousal and to reduce deviant sexual urges and behaviors in men with paraphilias. Indeed, Bourgeois & Klein (1996) recently described a 27-year-old man with pedophilia and dysthymic disorder unresponsive to fluoxetine monotherapy (80 mg/day) whose pedophilic and dysthymic symptoms responded completely when risperidone (6 mg/day) was added to the fluoxetine. By contrast, a double-blind, placebo-controlled comparison of the antopsychotic agents chlorpromazine and benperidal conducted by Tennent et al. (1974) in 12 male pedophilic offenders found that neither agent was superior to placebo in reducing measures of spontaneous sexual behaviors and penile erections in response to erotic stimuli. However, self-ratings of frequency of sexual thoughts were significantly lower on benperidal than on chlorpromazine or placebo.

Antidepressants: Antidepressant agents also affect sexual behavior in multiple ways. First, a wide range of antidepressant agents are associated with various types of sexual dysfunction (Balon et al., 1993; Gitlin 1994; Harrison et al., 1986; Montejo-Gonzalez et al., 1997). Examples of antidepressant - induced sexual dysfunction include decreased libido, impaired ejaculation, delayed orgasm, painful orgasm, anorgasmia, erectile dysfunction and priapism. In general, tricyclics, monoamine oxidase inhibitors, SRIs, and trazodone have been implicated more frequently in causing sexual dysfunction than have bupropion, nefazodone, and mirtazipine. Second, antidepressants may improve reduced libido and sexual dysfunction associated with depressive disorders. Third, as noted earlier, numerous case reports, several open studies, and two preliminary controlled trials suggest that antidepressants, including tricyclics and SRIs inhibitors, may be effective in reducing the deviant and excessive sexual fantasies and behaviors, respectively, of paraphilias and NPSAs (Federoff, 1993; Greenberg & Bradford, 1997; Kafka, 1994a, 1995; Kruesi et al., 1992; Zohar et al.,1994). Of note, these agents have been reported to be effective in persons with aggressive as well as nonaggressive paraphilias (Kafka, 1991b), and to reduce paraphilic symptoms without adversely affecting normal sexual function (Kafka, 1991a). In addition, SRIs reduce sexual obsessions of OCD, and in case reports, have been used successfully to treat hypersexual behavior associated with dementia (Stewart & Shin, 1997). Finally, virtually any antidepressant may exacerbate the abnormal sexual behavior associated with manic and mixed affective states.

Mood stabilizers: In general, the literature suggests that mood stabilizers, which include lithium, valproate, carbamazepine, and possibly the new antiepileptic drugs gabapentin, lamotrigine, and topiramate, have fewer adverse effects on sexual function than do the antipsychotics and antidepressants, though sexual dysfunction has been described for lithium (Ghadirian et al.,1992; Gitlin, 1994). Systematic studies comparing the sexual side effects of these agents, however, have not been conducted.

Mood stabilizers reduce abnormal sexual behavior associated with mania and mixed states. Moreover, there are isolated reports of lithium being effective in persons with paraphilias (e.g., transvestism, autoerotic asphyxiation) with and without comorbid bipolar disorder (Cesnik & Coleman 1989; Ward, 1975). There is also a report of carbamazepine being effective in a man with several paraphilias caused by both frontal and temporal lobe damage (Goldberg & Buongiorno, 1982–83).

Antiandrogens or testosterone-lowering medications: Both open (Kravitz et al., 1995; Meyer et al., 1992; Rösler & Witztum, 1998) and controlled (Bradford & Pawlak, 1993, Cooper, 1981; Cooper et al., 1992; Hucker et al., 1989; Wincze et al., 1986) studies suggest that hormonal agents that reduce testosterone function, such as medroxyprogesterone acetate (MPA)(which antagonizes the secretion of gonadotropin and thus of testosterone), cyproterone acetate (CPA)(which antagonizes testosterone function), and the gonadotropin-releasing hormone agonist (GnRH) analogues triptorelin and leuprolide acetate (LPA), decrease not only normal sex drive and function, but also deviant sexual thoughts, fantasies, and behaviors in men with paraphilias, including those convicted of sexual crimes (Abel & Osborn, 1995; Gijs & Gooren, 1996; Bradford, 1988; 1990, 1998). GnRH agonist analogues may be effective when MPA and/or CPA have failed. Moreover, there have also been reports that these agents may reduce irritability and other nonsexual aggressive behaviors in such persons. Indeed it has been suggested by some authorities that such drugs should be the medications of choice in the management of socially unacceptable sexual behavior (e.g., pedophilia, rape) in persons convicted of sexual crimes, especially if the patient also suffers from hypersexuality or aggressivity (Cooper et al., 1992).

The results of studies of antiandrogens in persons with abnormal sexual behavior, however, must be interpreted with caution (Richer & Crismon, 1993). Subjects were primarily sex offenders with paraphilias. Subjects in open trials were also receiving extensive psychosocial treatments for their paraphilias. Controlled trials with positive findings generally used small sample sizes. Not all controlled trials were positive. For example, a controlled, double-blind, within-subjects, crossover trial in which eight subjects received MPA or sterile saline in four alternating 16-week blocks over a 64-week period conducted by Kiersch (1990) found favorable results with both injected substances. Moreover, as noted earlier, treatment with these agents suppresses normal, as well as deviant, sexual drive and behavior, and is associated with numerous uncomfortable and some potentially dangerous side effects. For MPA, these include (in addition to sexual dysfunction): fatigue, weight gain, hepatic dysfunction, depression, leg cramps, hypertension, diabetes mellitus, cholecystitis with cholelithiasis, gynecomastia, thrombophlebitis, and pulmonary embolism. Indeed, some studies suggest that only a small proportion of persons with paraphilias are willing to accept treatment with these agents (Cooper et al., 1992).

Nonetheless, these agents are extremely important components of the therapeutic armamentarium for abnormal sexual behavior, particularly for aggressive hypersexuality or deviant sexual behavior (e.g., pedophilia, sexual sadism, and other aggressive paraphilias) that has failed to respond to more conventional pharmacologic treatments (e.g., antidepressants, mood stabilizers, and/or antipsychotics). Also, there are case reports of the successful use of these agents in the treatment of hypersexuality associated with schizophrenia (Cooper et al., 1990) and dementia (Cooper, 1987; Ott, 1995).

Opioid antagonists: As noted earlier, male erectile dysfunction has been reported to respond to the opioid antagonist naltrexone (Fabbri et al., 1989). To our knowledge, there are no studies of such agents in persons with hypersexuality or paraphilias. However, based on the similarities between paraphilias and NPSAs on the one hand and substance use and impulse control disorders on the other, the proven efficacy of naltrexone in alcohol dependence (O'Brien et al., 1996), and isolated reports of the successful use of naltrexone in various impulse control disorders (Kim, 1998), trials of opioid antagonists might be considered in persons with paraphilias and NPSAs resistant to thymoleptic and antiandrogen agents, particularly in those persons with comorbid alcohol use disorders.

IV. Assessment and Pharmacologic Treatment Recommendations

When evaluating any patient for abnormal sexual behavior, it is first important to be aware that this is an important issue that may not come to the clinician's attention unless the patient is directly and systematically asked about his or her sexual functioning and interests (also see Burkley et al., Chapter 1; and Deegan, Chapter 2). This requires open-ended questions about sexual functioning as well as direct questions about sexual desire, excitement, orgasm, masturbation, and types and frequencies of sexual fantasies, urges, and behaviors. For example, when evaluating for NPSAs, patients might initially be asked if they feel any of their sexual thoughts or behaviors are excessive or compulsive, or whether they feel addicted to any of their sexual thoughts or behaviors. When evaluating for paraphilias, patients might be initially asked if there is anything unusual or out of the ordinary which they find sexually stimulating or arousing. After open-ended questions, however, patients need to be asked about specific NPSAs and paraphilias.

When a patient identifies or admits to problematic sexual symptoms or behaviors, the patients must then be asked how wanted versus unwanted, impulsive versus compulsive, and pleasurable versus repulsive his or her sexual symptoms are to him or her. Patients must also be thoroughly evaluated for non-sexual Axis I disorders, including psychotic, mood, substance use, anxiety, eating, attention-deficit hyperactivity and impulse control disorders; Axis II disorders, especially cluster B disorders; degree of psychopathy and sadism; and whether they have any medical disorders or neurological deficits or are taking any medications or substances that might be contributing to their abnormal sexual behavior.

Based on this assessment, it should be determined whether pharmacologic treatment might be helpful in the management of the abnormal sexual behavior of that particular patient. Specifically, in patients with abnormal sexual thoughts or behaviors due to or accompanied by a psychotic, mood, or anxiety disorder, appropriate pharmacologic treatment for the underlying disorder is initiated. Thus, an antipsychotic (e.g., olanzapine, quetiapine, risperidone, or a typical antipsychotic) is begun for the patient with a psychotic disorder, a mood stabilizer (e.g., lithium, valproate, or carbamazepine) is begun for the patient with a bipolar disorder, an antidepressant is begun for the patient with a depressive disorder, and a serotonin reuptake inhibitor is begun for the patient with OCD with sexual obsessions.

For the person whose abnormal sexual ideation or behavior is due to a paraphilia or a NPSA, our initial pharmacologic treatment choice depends on whether that person has comorbid affective symptoms or a comorbid mood disorder. Specifically, for the person with either no comorbid mood disorder, comorbid depressive symptoms, or a comorbid depressive disorder (i.e., major depressive disorder or dysthymia), pharmacologic treatment is usually initiated with an SRI (e.g., fluoxetine, fluvoxamine, paroxetine, sertraline, or venlafaxine). For the person with comorbid hypomanic symptoms or a comorbid bipolar disorder (type I, II, or cyclothymia), treatment is usually initiated with a mood stabilizer, particularly if the person is actively displaying manic, hypomanic, mixed, or rapid cycling affective symptoms. Of note, if the latter patient displays mixed or rapid cycling symptoms as opposed to pure manic or hypomanic symptoms, we tend to choose valproate before lithium as first-line treatment because of studies demonstrating valproate's superior efficacy over lithium in mania associated with depressive symptoms (Swann *et al.*, 1997).

For the patient with a paraphilia or NPSA and a comorbid mood disorder, we closely follow the affective symptoms along with the sexual symptoms as we proceed with pharmacological treatment. Thus, for the patient with depressive and paraphilic symptoms who fails to respond adequately to the first antidepressant, we may augment the first agent if there has been a partial response (e.g., with a second SRI or even an atypical antipsychotic in the patient with prominent obsessive-compulsive or other anxiety disorder symptoms, or a norepinephrine reuptake inhibitor in the patient with comorbid attention-deficit disorder symptoms) or switch to a second agent (typically another SRI) if there has been no or minimal response. For the patient who displays persistent manic, hypomanic, or mixed affective symptoms despite treatment with a mood stabilizer, a second and sometimes a third mood stabilizer and/or an antipsychotic (e.g., olanzapine, quetiapine, a typical antipsychotic) is substituted for or added to the first or second mood stabilizer. If the patient becomes depressed and/or continues to experience paraphilic symptoms after adequate mood stabilizer treatment, an antidepressant (usually an SRI) is added to the mood stabilizer regimen. For the patient who develops hypomanic or manic symptoms with antidepressant treatment, the antidepressant is discontinued or reduced in dose, the mood stabilizer is increased in dose, and/or a second mood stabilizer and/ or an antipsychotic is added.

As noted earlier, for the patient with a paraphilia or NPSA and a comorbid mood disorder, we carefully assess the patients' sexual symptoms as his or her affective symptoms are stabilized. If the patient's sexual symptoms respond as his or her affective symptoms respond, we continue the effective thymoleptic regimen as maintenance therapy. However, if the patient's affective symptoms respond but his or her sexual symptoms persist, we consider augmentation therapy with other thymoleptics (e.g., adding an SRI to a mood stabilizer), antipsychotics (especially atypical agents), and/or antiandrogen agents (e.g., adding MPA or a GNRH agonist analogue to the thymoleptic regimen). If these strategies fail, we consider adjunctive treatment with an opiate antagonist, particularly if the patient has a comorbid substance use or impulse control disorder.

For the person with abnormal sexual behavior thought to be due to antisocial or borderline personality disorder and/or psychopathy, pharmalogic treatment is guided by the presence of associated affective (i.e., bipolar versus depressive) and/or impulsive versus compulsive features. Thus, we consider empirical trials of mood stabilizers (especially with the antiepileptic agents valproate and carbamazepine) for persons with prominent affective instability, lability, or irritability;

trials of SRIs for persons with prominent impulsivity, especially impulsive aggression, or obsessive-compulsive features; trials of antiandrogen agents for men with prominent hypersexuality, especially when associated with aggression and/or deviance; and trials of opiate antagonists for men with comorbid substance use disorders. We consider similar empirical trials for persons with abnormal sexual behavior due to or associated with brain damage and/or medical illness, including that from head trauma, dementia, and mental retardation. Non pharmacologic treatments and support are comprehensively covered by Kopelowitz and colleagues (Chapter 6) in this book.

V. CONCLUSION

In conclusion, abnormal sexual behavior, including sexual hypofunction or dysfunction, sexual hyperfunction, and deviant sexual behavior, is an important but underrecognized problem among persons with mental illness. Pharmacologic treatment is often helpful in the management of all types of abnormal sexual behavior. Careful elucidation of the nature, etiology, and comorbid psychiatric and medical features of the abnormal sexual behavior will aid in determining what that pharmacologic treatment should entail.

REFERENCES

Abel, G.G., Becker, J.V., Cunningham-Rathner, J., Mittelman, M. & Rouleau, J.-L. (1988). Multiple paraphilic diagnoses among sex offenders. *Bull Am Acad Psychiatry Law* 16:153–168.

Abel, G.G. & Osborn, C.A. (1995). Pedophilia. In: *Treatments of Psychiatric disorders. Second Edition.* (Ed. G.O. Gabbard). American Psychiatric Press, Washington, D.C., pp. 1959–1975.

American Psychiatric Association (1980). *Diagnostic and Statistical Manual of Mental Disorders, 3rd ed.* American Psychiatric Association, Washington, D.C.

American Psychiatric Association (1987). *Diagnostic and Statistical Manual, 3rd ed.- revised.* American Psychiatric Association, Washington, D.C.

American Psychiatric Association (1994). *Diagnostic and Statistical Manual of Mental Disorder, 4th ed.* American Psychiatric Association, Washington, D.C.

Anthony, D.T & Hollander, E. (1993). Sexual compulsions. In: Hollander, E. ed. *Obsessive-Compulsive Related Disorders*, American Psychiatric Press, Washington, D.C. pp. 139–150.

Balon, R., Yeragani, V.K., Pohl, R. & Ramesh, C. (1993). Sexual dysfunction during antidepressant treatment. *Journal of Clinical Psychiatry* 54: 209–212

Bancroft, J., Tennant, G., Loucas, K. & Cass, J. (1974). The control of deviant sexual behavior by drugs: I. Behavioral changes following oestrogens and anti-androgens. *British Journal of Psychiatry* 125:310–315.

Bartholomew, A.A. (1968). A long-acting phenothiazine as a possible agent to control deviant sexual behavior. *American Journal of Psychiatry* 124: 77–83.

Bell, D.S. & Trethowan, W.H. (1961). Amphetamine addiction and disturbed sexuality. *Archives of General Psychiatry* 4:74–78.

Black, D.W., Kehrberg, L.L.D., Flumerfelt, D.L. & Schlosser, S.S. (1997). Characteristics of 36 subjects reporting compulsive sexual behavior. *American Journal of Psychiatry* 154:243–249.

Boolell, M., Allen, M.J., Ballard, S.A., Gepi-Attee, S., Muirhead, G.J., Naylor, A. M., Osterloh, I.H. & Gingell, C. (1996a). Sildenafil: An orally active type 5 cyclic GMP-specific phosphodiesterase inhibitor for the treatment of penile erectile dysfunction. *International Journal of Impotence Research* 8:47–52.

Boolell, M., Gepi-Attee, S., Gingell, J.C. & Allen, M.J. (1996b). Sildenafil, a novel effective oral therapy for male erectile dysfunction. *British Journal of Urology* 78:257–261.

Bourgeois, J.A. & Klein, M. (1996). Risperidone and fluoxetine in the treatment of pedophilia with comorbid dysthymia. *Journal of Clinical Psychopharmacology* 16:257–258 (letter).

Bradford, J.M.W. (1988). Organic treatment for the male sexual offender. *Annals of New York Academy of Sciences* 528:193–202.

Bradford, J.M.W. (1990). The antiandrogen and hormonal treatment of sex offenders. In: *Handbook of Sexual Assault* (eds. Marshall, W.L., Laws, D.R. and Barbaree, H.E.) pp. 297–310. Plenum Press, New York.

Bradford, J.M.W. (1998). Treatment of men with paraphilias. *The New England Journal of Medicine* 338:464–465.

Bradford, J.M.W., Boulet, J. & Pawlak, A. (1992). The paraphilias: A multiplicity of deviant behaviors. *Canadian Journal of Psychiatry* 37:104–108.

Bradford, J.M.W. & Pawlak, A. (1993). A double-blind placebo crossover study of CPA in the treatment of the paraphilias. *Archives of Sexual Behavior* 22:383–402.

Carnes, P.J. (1990). Sexual addiction: progress, criticism, challenges. *American Journal of Preventative Psychiatry Neurology* 2:1–8.

Carrier, S., Brock, G., Kour, N.W. & Lue, T.F. (1993). Pathophysiology of erectile dysfunction. *Urology* 42:468–481.

Cesnik, J.A. & Coleman, E. (1989). Use of lithium carbonate in the treatment of autoerotic asphyxia. *American Journal of Psychotherapy* 63:277–286.

Coleman, E. (1987). Sexual compulsivity: Definition, etiology, and treatment considerations. *Journal of Chemical Dependency Treatment* 1:189–204.

Cooper, A.J. (1977). Bromocriptine in impotence. *Lancet* iii:567.

Cooper, A.J. (1981). A placebo-controlled trial of the antiandrogen cyproterone acetate in deviant hypersexuality. *Comprehensive Psychiatry* 22:458–465.

Cooper, A.J. (1987). Medroxyprogesterone acetate (MPA) treatment of sexual acting out in men suffering from dementia. *Journal of Clinical Psychiatry* 48:368–370.

Cooper, A.J., Ismail, A.A.A., Phanjoo, A.L. & Love, D.L. (1972). Antiandrogen (cyproterone acetate) therapy in deviant hypersexuality. *British Journal of Psychiatry* 120:59–63.

Cooper, A.J., Losftyn, S., Russell, N.C. & Cernovsky, F. (1990). Medroxyprogesterone acetate, nocturnal penile tumescence, laboratory arousal, and sexual acting out in a male with schizophrenia. *Archives of Sexual Behavior* 19:361–372.

Cooper, A.J., Sandhu, S., Losztyn, S. & Cernovsky, F. (1992). A double-blind placebo controlled trial of medroxyprogesterone acetate and cyproterone acetate with seven pedophiles. *Canadian Journal of Psychiatry* 37:687–693.

Croughan, J.L., Saghir, M., Cohne, R. & Robins, E. (1981). A comparison of treated and untreated male cross-dressers. *Archives of Sexual Behavior* 10:515–528.

Everitt, B.J. (1983). Monoamines and the control of sexual behavior. *Psychological Medicine* 13:715–720.

Eyres, A. (1960). Transvestism: Employment of somatic therapy with subsequent improvement. *Diseases Nervous System* 21:52–53.

Fabbri, A., Jannini, E., Gnessi, L., Moretti, S., Ulisse, S., Franzese, A., Lazzari, R., Fraioli, F., Frajese, G. & Isidori, A. (1989). Endorphins in male impotence: Evidence for Naltrexone stimulation of erectile activity in patient therapy. *Psychoneuroendocrinology* 14:103–111.

Federoff, J. (1988). Buspirone hydrochloride in the treatment of transvestic fetishism. *Journal of Clinical Psychiatry* 48:408–409.

Federoff, J.P. (1993). Serotonergic drug treatment of deviant sexual interests. *Annals of Sex Research* 6:105–121.

Federoff, J.P., Peyser, C., Franz, M.L. & Folstein, S.E. (1994). Sexual disorders in Huntington's disease. *Journal of Neuropsychiatry and Clinical Neurosciences* 6:147–153.

Fedora, O., Reddon, J.R., Morrison, J.W., Fedora, S.K., Pascoe, H. & Yeudall, L.T. (1992). Sadism and other paraphilias in normal controls and aggressive and nonaggressive sex offenders. *Archives of Sexual Behavior* 21:1–15.

Feighner, J., Robins, E., Guze, S.B. *et al.* (1972). Diagnostic criteria for use in psychiatric research. *Archives of General Psychiatry* 16:57–63.

Gagne, P. (1981). Treatment of sex offenders with medroxyprogesterone acetate. *American Journal of Psychiatry* 138:644–646.

Galli, V., McElroy, S.L., Soutullo, C.A., Kizer, D., Raule, N., Keck, P.E., Jr. & McConville, B. (1999). The psychiatric diagnoses of twenty-two adolescents who have sexually molested other children. *Comprehensive Psychiatry* 40:85.

Gessa, G.L. & Tagliamonte, A. (1975). Role of brain serotonin and dopamine in male sexual behavior In: *Sexual Behavior: Pharmacology and Biochemistry* (eds Sandler, M. and Gessa, G.L.). Raven Press, New York.

Ghadirrian, A.M., Annable, L. & Bilanger, M.C. (1992). Lithium, benzodiazepines, and sexual function in bipolar patients. *American Journal of Psychiatry* 149:801–805.

Girgis, S.M., El-Haggen, S. & El-Hermouzy, S. (1982). A double blind trial of clomipramine in premature ejaculation. *Andrologia* 14:364–368.

Gitlin, M. (1994). Psychotropic medications and their effects on sexual function: diagnosis, biology, and treatment approaches. *Journal of Clinical Psychiatry* 55:406–413.

Goldberg, R.L. & Buongiorno, P.A. (1982–83). The use of carbamazepine for the treatment of paraphilias in a brain damaged patient. *International Journal Psychiatry in Medicine* 12:275–279.

Goldstein, I., Lue, T.F., Padma-Nathan, H., Rosen, R.C., Steers, W.D. & Wickers, P.A. for the sildenafil study Group. (1998). Oral sildenafil in the treatment of erectile dysfunction. *New England Journal of Medicine* 338:1397–1404.

Goodman, R.E. (1980). An assessment of clomipramine (Anafranil) in the treatment of premature ejaculation. *Journal of International Medical Research* 8:(suppl 3), 53–59.

Goodwin, F.K. & Jamison, K.R. (1990). *Manic-Depressive Illness.* Oxford University Press, New York.

Gottesman, H.G. & Schubert, D.S. (1993). Low-dose oral medroxyprogesterone acetate in the management of paraphilias. *Journal of Clinical Psychiatry* 54:182–188.

Greenberg, D.M. & Bradford, J.M.W. (1997). Treatment of the paraphilic disorders: A review of the role of the selective serotonin reuptake inhibitors. *Sexual abuse: A Journal of Research and Treatment* 9:349–360.

Gregoire, A. (1992). New treatments for erectile impotence. *British Journal of Psychiatry* 160:315–326.

Harrison, W.M., Rabkin, J.G., Ehrhardt, A.A., Stewart, J.W., McGrath, P.J., Ross, D. & Quitkin, F.M. (1986). Effects of antidepressant medication on sexual function: a controlled study. *Journal of Clinical Psychopharmacology* 6:144–149.

Henn, R.A., Herjanic, M. & Vanderpearl, R.H. (1976). Forensic psychiatry: Profiles of two types of sex offenders. *American Journal of Psychiatry* 133:694–696.

Hollander, E. (1993). Obsessive-Compulsive Related Disorders. Washington, D.C: American Psychiatric Press.

Hollander, E. & Wong, C.M. (1995). Body dysmorphic disorder, pathological gambling, and sexual compulsions. *Journal of Clinical Psychiatry* 56 [Suppl 4] 7–12.

Hucker, S., Langevin, R., Dickey, R., Handy, L., Chambers, J. & Wright, S. (1988). Cerebral damage and dysfunction in sexually aggressive men. *Annals of Sex Research* 1:33–47.

Hucker, S.J., Langevin, J. & Bain, J. (1989) A double-blind trial of sex drive reducing medication in pedophiles. *Annals of Sex Research* 1: 227–242.

Kafka, M.P. (1991a). Successful antidepressant treatment of nonparaphilic sexual addictions and paraphilias in men. *Journal of Clinical Psychiatry* 52:60–65.

Kafka, M.P. (1991b). Successful treatment of paraphilic coercive disorder (a rapist) with fluoxetine hydrochloride. *British Journal of Psychiatry* 158:844–847.

Kafka, M.P. (1994a). Paraphilia-related disorders – common, neglected and misunderstood. *Harvard Review of Psychiatry* 2:39–40.

Kafka, M.P. (1994b). Sertraline pharmacotherapy for paraphilias and paraphilias and paraphilia-related disorders: an open trial. *Annals of Clinical Psychiatry*.

Kafka, M.P. (1995). Sexual impulsivity. In: Impulsivity and Aggression (Eds. Hollander, E. and Stein, D.J.). John Wiley & Sons, Chicester, England, pp. 201–228.

Kafka, M.P. & Prentky, R. A. (1992a). A comparative study of nonparaphilic sexual addictions and paraphilias in men. *Journal of Clinical Psychiatry* 53:345–350.

Kafka, M.P. & Prentky, R. (1992b). Fluoxetine treatment of nonparaphilic sexual addictions and paraphilias in men. *Journal of Clinical Psychiatry* 53:351–358.

Kafka, M.P. & Prentky, R. A. (1994). Preliminary observations of DSM-IV Axis I comorbidity in men with paraphilias and paraphilia-related disorders. *Journal of Clinical Psychiatry* 55:481–487.

Kane, J.M. & Lieberman, J.A. (Eds). (1992). Adverse Effects of Psychotropic Drugs. The Guilford Press, New York.

Kaplan, H.S. (1995). Sexual desire disorders (hypoactive sexual desire and sexual aversion). In: *Treatments of Psychiatric Disorders. Second edition.* (Ed G.O. Gabbard). American Psychiatric Press, Washingon, D.C., pp. 1843–1866.

Kiersch, T.A. (1990). Treatment of sex offenders with Depo-Provera. *Bulletin of the American Academy of Psychiatry and the Law* 18:179–187.

Kim, S.W. (1998). Opioid antagonists in the treatment of impulse control disorders. *Journal of Clinical Psychiatry* 59:159–164.

Kravitz, H.M., Haywood, T.W., Kelly, J., Wahlstrom, C., Liles, S. & Cavanaugh, J.L.Jr. (1995). Medroxyprogesterone treatment for paraphiliacs. *Bulletin of the American Academy of Psychiatry and the Law* 23: 19–33.

Kruesi, M.J.P., Fine, S., Valladares, L., Philips, R.A. & Rapaport, J.L. (1992). Paraphilias: A double-blind crossover comparison of clomipramine versus desipramine. *Archives of Sexual Behavior* 21:587–593.

Lal, S., Tesfaye, Y., Thavundayil, J.K., Thompson, T.R., Kiely, M.E., Nair, N.P., Grassimo, A. & Dubovsky, B. (1989). Apomorphine: Clinical studies on erectile impotence and yawning. *Neuro-Psychopharmalogical and Biological Psychiatry* 13:329–339.

MacCullouch, M.J., Snowden, P.R., Wood, P.J.W. & Mills, H.E. (1983). Sadistic fantasy, sadistic behavior and offending. *British Journal of Psychiatry* 14434:20–29.

Maletzky, B.M. (1991) *Treating the Sexual Offender.* Sage Publications, Newbury Park, CA.

Mann, K., Klinger, T., Now, S., Roschke, J., Muller, S. & Benkert, O. (1996). Effects of yohimbine on sexual experiences and nocturnal penile tumescence and rigidity in erectile dysfunctions. *Archives of Sexual Behavior* 25:1–16.

McElroy, S.L., Hudson, J.I., Phillips, K.A., Keck, P.E. Jr. & Pope, H.G. Jr. (1993). Clinical and theoretical implications of a possible link between obsessive-compulsive and impulse control disorders. *Depression* 1:121–132.

McElroy, S.L., Keck, P.E., Jr, Hudson, J.I., Phillips, K.A. & Strakowski, S.M. (1996). Are impulse control disorders related to bipolar disorder? *Comprehensive Psychiatry* 37:229–240.

Meloy, J.R. (1997). The psychology of wickedness: Psychopathy and sadism. *Psychiatric Annals* 27:630–633.

Meyer III, W.J., Cole, C. & Emory, E. (1992). Depo-Provera treatment for sex offending behavior: An evaluation of outcome. *Bulletin of the American Academy of Psychiatry and the Law* 20:249–259.

Montejo-Gonzalez, A.L., Liorca, G., Izquierdo, J.A., Ledesma, A., Bousono, M., Calcedo, A., Carrasco, J.L., Crudad, J., Daniel, E., De La Gandara, J., Franco, M., Gomez, M.J., Marcias, J.A., Martin, T., Perez, V., Sanchez, J.M., Sanchez, S. & Vicens, E. (1997). SSRI-induced sexual dysfunction: Fluoxetine, paraxetine, sertraline, and fluvoxamine in a prospective, multicenter, and descriptive clinical study of 344 patients. *Journal of Sex and Marital Therapy* 23:176–193.

Morales Ott, B.R. (1995). Leuprolide treatment of sexual aggression in a patient with dementia and the Kluver-Bucy syndrome. *Clinical Neuropharmacology* 18:443–447.

Nelson, E.B., Keck, P.E. Jr. & McElroy, S.L. (1997). Resolution of fluoextine induced sexual dysfunction with the 5HT-3 antagonist granisetron. *Journal of Clinical Psychiatry* 58:496–497.

O'Brien, C.P., Volpicelli, L.A. & Volpicelli, J.R. (1996). Naltrexone in the treatment of alcoholism: A clinical review. *Alcohol* 13:35–39.

O'Carroll R. & Bancroft, J. (1984) Testosterone therapy for low sexual interest and erectile dysfunction in men: a controlled study. *British Journal of Psychiatry* 145:146–151.

O'Carroll, R., Shapiro C. & Bancroft, J. (1985). Androgens, behavior and nocturnal erection in hypogonadal men: The effects of varying replacement dose. *Clinical Endocrinology* 23:527–538.

O'Donohue, W. & Geer, J.H. (1993). *Handbook of Sexual Dysfunctions.* Needham Heights, MA: Simon & Schuster.

Pearson, H.J. (1990). Paraphilias, impulse control, and serotonin. *Journal of Clinical Psychopharmacology* 10:223 (letter).

Perilstein, R.D., Lipper, S. & Friedman, L.J. (1991). Three cases of paraphilias responsive to fluoxetine treatment. *Journal of Clinical Psychiatry* 52: 169–170.

Pope, H.G. & Katz, D.L. Psychiatric effects of exogenous anabolic-androgenic steroids. In: *Psychoneuroendocrinology for the Clinician.* (Eds. O.M. Wolkowitz and A.J. Rothschild). American Psychiatric Press, Washington, D.C., In press.

Rabkin, R. & Wagner, G. (1995). Testosterone replacement in HIV illness. *General Hospital Psychiatry* 17:37–42.

Reid, K., Surridge, D.H.C., Morales, A., Condra, M. & Harris, C. (1987). Double-blind trial of yohimbine in treatment of psychogenic impotence. *Lancet* 2:421–423.

Richer, M. & Crismon, M.L. (1993). Pharmacotherapy of sexual offenders. *Annals of Pharmacotherapy* 27:316–320.

Riley, A.J., Goodman, R.E., Kellet, J.M. & Orr, R. (1989). Double-blind trial of yohimbine hydrochloride in the treatment of erection inadequacy. *Sex and Marital Therapy* 4:17–26.

Rösler, A. & Witztum, E. (1998). Treatment of men with paraphilia with a long acting analogue of gonadotropin-releasing hormone. *The New England Journal of Medicine* 338:416–422.

Schiavi, R.C. (1995). Male erectile disorder. In: *Treatments of Psychiatric Disorders. Second Edition.* (Ed G.O. Gabbard). American Psychiatric Press, Washington, D.C., pp. 1867–1885.

Segraves, R.T. (1989). Effects of psychotropic drugs on human erection and ejaculation. *Archives of General Psychiatry* 46:275–284.

Stein, D.J., Hollander, E., Anthony, D.T., Schneier, F. R., Fallon, B.A., Liebowitz, R.W. & Klein, D.F. (1992). Serotonergic medications for sexual obsessions, sexual addictions, and paraphilias. *Journal of Clinical Psychiatry* 53:267–271.

Stewart, J.T. & Shin, K.J. (1997). Paroxetine treatment of sexual disinhibition in dementia. *American Journal of Psychiatry* 154:1474 (letter).

Susset, J.G., Tessier, C.D., Wincze, J, Bansal, S., Malhotra, C. & Schwacha, M.G. (1989). Effect of yohimbine hydrochloride on erectile impotence : A double-blind study. *Journal of Urology* 141:1360–1363.

Swann, A.C., Bowden, C.L. Morris, D., Calabrese, J.R., Petty, F., Small, J., Dilsaver, S.C. & Davis, J.M. (1997). Depression during mania. Treatment response to lithium or divalproex. *Archives of General Psychiatry* 54: 37–42.

Tennant, G., Bancroft, J. & Cass, J. (1974). The control of deviant sexual behavior by drugs: A double-blind controlled study of haloperidol, chlorpromazine, and placebo. *Archives of Sexual Behavior* 3:261–271.

Terrett, N.K., Bell, A.S., Brown, D. & Ellis, P. (1996). Sildenafil (VigraTM), a potent and selective inhibitor of type 5 CGMP phosphodiesterase with utility for the treatment of male erectile dysfunction. *Bioorganic & Medicinal Chemistry Letters* 6:1819–1824.

Virkkunen, M. (1985). The pedophilic offender with antisocial character. *Acta Psychiatrica Scandinavica* 53:401–405.

Waldinger, M.D., Hengereld, M.W. & Fwinderman, A.H.(1994). Paroxetine treatment of premature ejaculation: A double-blind, randomized, placebo-controlled study. *American Journal of Psychiatry* 151:1377–1379.

Ward, N.G. (1975). Successful lithium treatment of transvestism associated with manic depression. *Journal of Nervous and Mental Disease* 161:204–206.

Wincze, J.P., Bansal, S. & Malamud, M. (1986). Effects of medroxyprogesterone acetate on subjective arousal to erotic stimulation, and nocturnal penile tumescence in male sexual offenders. *Archives of Sexual Behavior* 15:193–305.

Young, R.L., Schreiber, M.T. & Nysewander, R.W. (1983). Psychotic mania. *Biological Psychiatry* 18:1167–1173.

Zohar, J., Kaplan, Z. & Benjamon, J. (1994). Compulsive exhibitionism successfully treated with fluoxamine: A controlled case study. *Journal of Clinical Psychiatry* 55:86–88.

Zubenko, G.S., George, A.W., Soloff, P.H. & Schulz, P. (1987). Sexual practices among patients with borderline personality disorder. *American Journal of Psychiatry* 144:748–752.

11

Sexuality, Stigma Busting and Mental Illness

PETER F. BUCKLEY and
THOMAS G. GUTHEIL

Individual chapters have addressed here several diverse aspects of human sexuality and mental illness: overall, however, the normality of human sexuality and, thereupon, the appropriateness of sexual expression in persons with serious mental illness emerges as the unifying theme of this book. The stance of 'benign neglect' – that is, feigned professional ignorance of the needs and occurrence of sexuality in persons with mental illness – is no longer tenable. Moreover, this denial of sexuality is blatantly unrealistic since it is now clear that persons suffering with mental illness do and will become sexually active. Despite these observations, three major concerns still conspire to uphold the position of benign neglect.

First, it is a truism, but no less important to state, that the recognition of sexuality in outpatients requires us to confront our own sexuality, both at a personal level and also in consideration of prevailing socio-sexual mores. Our training as mental health clinicians, particularly in latter years when psychodynamic principles have received less attention, discourages personalized reflection on patient issues. We are taught to be empathic, yet neutral. We are taught conscientiously to avoid intrusion of personal conflicts which could obfuscate the clinical circumstance. It is also implicit that, as clinicians treating abnormal mental health, we are somehow endowed with and knowledgeable about normal emotions. All of us have suffered the ignominy of being quizzed at a dinner party about some aspect of human intimacy as if we had (as regular psychiatrists) authored the best-selling paperback on 'the meaning of life'! It is perhaps, then, not surprising that we choose the more comfortable option of feigned ignorance of patient sexuality.

Is it acceptable for a 45-year old male resident of a long-stay facility to masturbate 6 times a week? And with what degree of privacy? Should persons who develop friendships as inpatients have the right to use or have access to private rooms for sexual expression? Are same-sex relationships acceptable for patients while in hospital? It seems inconceivable that these questions could be adequately answered without recourse to an exploration of one's own sexual identity and more. Additionally, our society is always confused on sexual matters. People tend to hold highly polarized opinions on fundamental aspects of sexuality. Are autoeroticism and masturbation immoral? At what age and in what mental states is sex consensual? Why is homosexuality ridiculed and feared by many? What is all the Viagra hype about? The complexity of human sexuality and the observed awkwardness of this topic when presented to the treatment team (what if the treating psychiatrist is homosexual and other staff are unaware of this?) are powerful obstacles which serve to keep open discussion of sexuality as a low priority topic.

If our human frailties on this topic can be appreciated by clinicians, then an agenda for dialogue can be set. Outside the treatment team meeting, clinicians should have a forum for open discussion of (patient) sexuality. This should, of course, have been preceded by formal teaching (and discussion) at an undergraduate and/or postgraduate level. Furthermore, in long-stay psychiatric facilities and group homes where sexual expression may be more manifest, staff should receive some training and sensitization to this issue during their initial orientation. Clinicians should receive explicit training on how to inquire about the details of a person's sexual life. Psychiatrists should, as Dr. Deegan exhorts, inquire regularly of their patients about the sexual side-effects of prescribed medications and they should be prepared to make treatment adjustments thereupon. Currently, most programs offer little or no direction to clinicians on these matters. Moreover, there is no consensus as to how best – and in what forum – this topic should be addressed among clinicians. It seems only reasonable that clinicians should receive exposure to and guidance on these matters *before* they inflict their own prejudices upon patients. Additionally, clarifying the educational needs of clinicians is a prerequisite to undertaking psychoeducational activities for persons with mental illness.

The preceding chapters have also highlighted some more concrete, but no less serious, deficiencies in our care. Persons with mental illness should have ease of access to professional advice on contraception. They should receive education on sexuality, dating and relationships. They should, like the public at large, be informed on safe sex practices and have an awareness of the risk factors for sexually transmitted diseases. It is important however, as Drs. McKinnon and Cournos emphasize, to realize that simply acquiring information will not de facto effect behavioral change.

Second, sensitivity to all of the above issues is predicated upon a broader appreciation of the human potential of persons with mental illness. Essentially, social resistance to the combination of sexuality and mental illness can be subsumed under the larger topic of stigmatization of the mentally ill. The public and all too often the staff can no more easily imagine sexual relations among persons with mental illness than they can recognize sex between their own parents. In the eyes of many, it simply is not right. Moreover, as Dr. Deegan notes, the fear of mental illness and its perpetuation through transmission of genetic risk is always lurking in the public mind. So too is the stereotypic notion that sexual aberrance is associated with mental illness. Atrocities such as the notorious Jeffrey Dahmer case or the on-camera portrayal of mental and sexual aberrance in *Silence of the Lambs* sustain the public perception that raw and uncontrollable expression of the human drives of sex and aggression are manifested as an integral part of mental illness. To accept that individuals with mental illness may achieve human intimacy is to step outside a narrow medical model and to validate human potential. More complex models of care, such as the recovery model, accentuate this potential for fulfillment in persons with mental illness. At the present time, the focus of the National Alliance for the Mentally Ill's destigmatization campaign is the idea that mental illnesses are neurologic brain disorders. Paradoxically, this fine campaign may heighten public understanding at one level while drawing attention away from broader needs of persons with mental illness. The agenda for changing public opinion about mental illness is long, and more complex issues such as sexuality should, it could be argued, wait until the public has attained a broader appreciation of mental health issues. On the other hand, sexuality is such a fundamental issue that current public debate about mental illness may catalyze changes in perception that go well beyond these sexual matters. Consequently, discussion of sexual expression and mental illness must be sensible and must occur in the context of broader social and epidemiological considerations. Failure to do so could result in further public stigma and accusations that the mentally ill (through inadequate use of safe-sex practices) are vehicles for sexually transmitted diseases. Also, offering support for inpatient sexuality such as providing a privacy room, has been viewed as tantamount to prostitution-by-proxy.

Third, in some sense, the public interest in competency and personal freedom of choice together with, specifically, the passing of the ADA law have heightened medicolegal concerns around sexuality between patients. Fear of litigation has, in collision with benign neglect and stigmatization, been a major factor in sustaining the "don't ask, don't tell, don't discuss..." approach. At the present time, sex between persons in hospital may at best be private but it is rarely secret. Patients talk, staff talk, and a subculture exists in many long-stay facilities, a reality which gives double messages to patients. For example, hospital regulations stipulate "no sex", yet condoms are distributed upon request. Hospital responses are reactionary and the policy, if available, may be more applicable to extreme circumstances (such as inpatient rape) than to the prevailing issues. Fear of litigation and the need to protect vulnerable individuals is often in irreconcilable conflict with advocacy for personal autonomy. It is also important to appreciate that the law itself, about which people are always worried in this realm, is internally inconsistent in its ethical tensions between questions of freedom, protection and autonomy.

Information on hospital policies has already been covered in 2 chapters of this book and comments here will be brief. At a minimum, inpatient facilities which treat persons with mental illness should have some policy or guidelines regarding sexuality. It is unclear whether these should be generic enough to address all patient populations and circumstances or, alternatively, whether they should be selective and tailored to the population within that service. The prudence of having an inpatient policy or guidelines seems beyond debate. However, should policies for acute hospitals differ (e.g., have a total or time-limited prohibition on any sexual expression) from long-stay facilities? Also, do different issues apply for inpatient versus outpatient or are we obliged to take the position that it's all the same because of the overriding consideration of patient vulnerability? How restrictive should such policies be? This medicolegal responsibility for patient protection may also be greater where another patient is well known to engage in predatory behavior.

As this issue slips beyond the clinician into the administrative and public realms, its complexity and inconsistencies are intensified. Services are well advised at least to address this issue. However, it is also appropriate to advocate for a larger forum where various stakeholders may discuss this issue and formulate a consensus or blueprint policy which could be further modified by individual mental health systems and facilities. It is our hope that this book may be a beneficial contribution to such discussion.

Index